T0195426

2nd EDITION

Motor Assessment of the Developing Infant

Alberta Infant Motor Scale (AIMS)

Martha C. Piper, PhD
President Emeritus
University of British Columbia
Vancouver, British Columbia
Canada

Johanna Darrah, PhD
Professor Emerita
Faculty of Rehabilitation Medicine
University of Alberta
Edmonton, Alberta
Canada

Alicia Spittle, PhD
Associate Editor
Department of Physiotherapy
University of Melbourne
Clinical Sciences, Murdoch Children's Research Institute
Department of Physiotherapy,
The Royal Women's Hospital
Australia

ELSEVIER

ELSEVIER

3251 Riverport Lane
St. Louis, Missouri 63043

MOTOR ASSESSMENT OF THE DEVELOPING INFANT, SECOND EDITION

Previous edition copyrighted 1994.

Library of Congress Control Number: 2021940905

Content Strategist: Lauren Willis
Content Development Specialist: Kathleen Nahm
Publishing Services Manager: Deepthi Unni
Project Manager: Haritha Dharmarajan
Design Direction: Patrick Ferguson

Printed in the United States of America

Last digit is the print number: 9 8 7 6 5 4 3

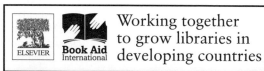

CONTRIBUTORS

Gayatri Kembhavi, PhD
Director
Centre for Evidence and Implementation
Singapore

Tom Maguire, PhD
Professor Emeritus
University of Alberta
Edmonton, Alberta
Canada

Lynn Redfern, PhD
Clinical Nurse Researcher (Ret.)
Edmonton, Alberta
Canada

Alicia Spittle, PhD
Department of Physiotherapy
University of Melbourne, Clinical
    Sciences
Murdoch Children's Research Institute,
    Department of Physiotherapy
The Royal Women's Hospital

ACKNOWLEDGMENTS

We are grateful to the individuals who contributed to this edition of the *Motor Assessment of the Developing Infant*:

Dr. Alicia Spittle, Professor at the University of Melbourne, and Associate Editor of this revision. Dr. Spittle is the lead author on Chapter 2, sharing her knowledge of infant motor development and test measurement. She reviewed all the revised chapters and provided valuable feedback. We thank her for sharing both her knowledge and her time.

Dr. Gayatri Kembhavi, Director, Centre for Evidence and Implementation in Singapore, coauthored Chapter 1. During her graduate studies at the University of Alberta, Gayatri worked as Project Coordinator for two longitudinal research projects using the AIMS and contributed to our understanding of the trajectory of infant gross motor skills.

Dr. Lynn Redfern and Dr. Tom Maguire updated Chapter 10 to include the predictive validity information. It was a delight to reconnect with them.

Taryn Barry, a doctoral student at the University of Alberta, read the chapters for clarity, reference styling, and typographical errors. We appreciate her attention to detail.

We also acknowledge the photographer Neil Boyce, whose original photos remain in this edition. His ability to see the item descriptors made the items come to life.

Most important, we thank all of the infants, their parents and caregivers, and therapists who have contributed to the development of the AIMS over the years by either being assessed or by using the AIMS when assessing the motor development of infants. Since the original publication of the AIMS thousands of families and their infants internationally have participated in AIMS research. Most of them volunteered for longitudinal projects requiring multiple assessments, both in their homes and at academic institutions. We thank them for their support and their endorsement of the AIMS.

Martha C. Piper, PhD
Johanna Darrah, PhD

PREFACE FOR THE FIRST EDITION

The human child is the greatest miracle of creation. Every single child, moreover, is a world of subtle secrets, a personality, a unique occurrence, never to be repeated on this earth.

Alva Myrdal, as quoted by Sissela Bok in Alva Myrdal, A Daughter's Memoir, Radcliff Biography Series, 1991 (p. 129)

As Sissela Bok highlights in her biography of her extraordinary mother, Nobel Prize winner Alva Myrdal, the relationships between parents and children are constantly changing. Roles, expectations, and needs continue to evolve, changing with age and time. Infants become children; children become adults; adults become parents; parents become children. Nothing is certain, nothing is static, nothing is predictable. Such is the case with child development in general and infant motor development in particular.

The splendor of infancy is perhaps best expressed and celebrated by observing the infant explore and discover the world through the development of movement. The demonstrable skill of movement provides tangible evidence that the infant is evolving, becoming a personality, a unique occurrence. As with the infant's personality, the ability to move against gravity and assume an upright position evolves and matures. While movement unfolds, to a large extent in a predictable fashion, the subtleties each child brings to the process ensure that no two infants are exactly alike in how they move or evolve.

To witness the unfolding of motor skills during an infant's first 2 years of life contributes to the sense of wonder surrounding infant development. During these months, the motor abilities of an infant explode, so much that often it is difficult to absorb all the changes that occur. The rate of change in early motor development presents a special challenge to health care professionals involved in the assessment of infants' motor skills. Any assessment of motor skills in infancy is limited by the fact that we are forced to make a static evaluation of a dynamic process. The evolution of motor skills is a fluid, changing phenomenon, displaying many different facets that are dependent on the interaction of a myriad of variables. Factors as diverse as the motivation of the infant, the environment, the time of day, and the presence of a stranger may influence how an infant moves. When viewed from this perspective, any one evaluation of motor abilities is only an estimation of an infant's skills.

By observing the movements of over 2000 infants, all unique occurrences, we are convinced more than ever that what we do not know about infant movement far exceeds what we do know. Many aspects of motor development continue to elude us: Is motor development linear or continuous, or are there ebbs and flows in the normal unfolding of motor competency? Do early motor delays portend future motor deficits, or can an infant spontaneously "catch up"? Why do some infants choose not to creep on their hands and knees? What are the prerequisites for early walking?

Despite these unanswered questions, we are convinced that "knowing" about movement in infancy is far less important than "observing" movement in infancy. The infants have continued to surprise us with their "subtle secrets" and their ability to teach us about movement, rather than the other way around.

We are grateful to our teachers. As students, we find once again that our roles are reversed. The infants are instructing us, becoming parentlike in their abilities to inform us about the secrets of movement. We have become the children, in awe of our teachers, learning from their movements, their adaptations, and their creativeness.

And so we thank all of the infants who have contributed to this undertaking and who have so graciously shared their experiences with us. More than anything they have taught us to take the cues from them, to permit them to exhibit their unique strengths and abilities, and to celebrate their ability to discover and execute the movement required by their environments.

Martha C. Piper, PhD
Johanna Darrah, MSc, PT

The second edition of *Motor Assessment of the Developing Infant,* the manual for the Alberta Infant Motor Scale (AIMS), presents an opportunity to update and revise some content areas and to include research on the AIMS completed after the initial publication in 1994. Chapters 1 and 2 have been rewritten to reflect current thinking regarding how infant motor skills appear and change over time (Chapter 1), and the factors therapists need to consider when assessing infant motor abilities (Chapter 2). The clinical uses of the AIMS discussed in Chapter 9 have been updated with case examples; Chapter 10 includes a summary of the predictive validity study completed after publication of the first edition. The results of a reevaluation of the normative data are described in Chapter 11. Collectively these changes and additions reflect the "maturation" of both the AIMS and clinical reasoning in the area of infant gross motor skills.

An important addition to this edition is the development of an electronic scoresheet. Electronic medical records are becoming standard practice, and we have received many requests for an electronic version of the scoresheet. The print version of the scoresheet will continue to be available; users of the AIMS appreciate its "panoramic" view of gross motor skills, especially when discussing an infant's gross motor development with parents or caregivers.

The 58 items of the scale and the interpretative data in the appendices remain unchanged. The figures, item descriptors, and photographs of the 58 items have not been revised (Chapters 5–8). We made this decision for two different but equally important reasons. First, the psychometric properties of the AIMS are robust, and any changes to the items would require a reevaluation of the scale's reliability and validity. Second, the format of an AIMS assessment works well. We continue to receive feedback from users of the AIMS that they appreciate the observational approach of an AIMS assessment, the ease of scoring, and the use of the percentile graph and normative data to interpret an infant's performance. Users of the AIMS (and parents) often comment on how well the photographs capture the postures they observe when assessing an infant's motor skills.

We remember how pleased we were to see the items come to life in the photographer's studio. By the end of the 3-day shoot even the photographer started "seeing" the items. As the AIMS has aged, so too have the infants in the photographs who are now young adults. From its birth a quarter century ago, the AIMS has grown to become an established measure used to document the maturation of infant gross motor skills and is employed internationally as a research, clinical, and educational tool.

We are delighted to welcome Professor Alicia Spittle as Associate Editor of this second edition. As an early adopter of the AIMS, she attended one of the first presentations of the AIMS in Australia 16 years ago and later volunteered her infant son to be an assessment model at a subsequent AIMS training course. Since then she has become an internationally recognized leader in the areas of infant assessment measures and infant intervention programs and shares her knowledge globally through her research, clinical, and educational endeavors. We look forward to her continued involvement with the AIMS.

We have retained the original Preface. The quote from Alva Myrdal and our reflections at that time still capture our views about the emergence and maturation of infant motor skills. Despite changing theoretical perspectives, the publication of new infant motor measures, and increased knowledge of measurement issues, clinicians assessing infants' motor maturation are still surprised and sometimes puzzled by the infants' movement choices and eventual outcomes. The infants remain the teachers, and we, their students, learning from the "subtle secrets" they occasionally display. What we know about infant motor development is clearly less than what we don't know, thereby making the journey of observing infant motor skills extremely interesting, challenging, and never boring. We hope that the Alberta Infant Motor Scale continues to be a guide and a map for your personal journey of discovering the intricacies and delights of infant motor development.

Martha C. Piper, PhD
Johanna Darrah, PhD

CONTENTS

Motor Assessment of the Developing Infant

of the

Developing Infant

Alberta Infant Motor Scale (AIMS)

Theories of Motor Development

Johanna Darrah, Gayatri Kembhavi

An infant is born, and the journey of documenting developmental changes begins. Families celebrate and record a series of firsts—first smile, first roll, first tooth, first step. When these milestones appear at the expected age, it is confirmation that their infant is developing as anticipated. For parents[1] of infants with an increased risk of developmental challenges, the appearance of these firsts at the expected time is affirmation that their child is developing appropriately for their age. It is also important to identify if an infant is not reaching milestones within the expected age range so that families can be supported.

Infants at risk for developmental concerns are followed closely during their first 2 years to identify delays and, if necessary, to initiate early intervention programs to support the infant and family. Members of neonatal follow-up clinics (neonatologists, pediatricians, nurses, physical therapists, and occupational therapists) monitor the motor abilities of infants attending follow-up programs.[2] Gross motor milestones provide one of the earliest windows into an infant's developmental progress. To identify atypical motor development, therapists require an in-depth knowledge of typical motor development. Requiring more than a developmental checklist of motor skills, therapists need to understand the theoretical frameworks used to explain the *process* of development, in addition to the *output* of developmental maturation. A theoretical framework provides an explanation of how motor skills appear, and change can assist in the design of intervention programs to encourage the development of more mature motor skills.

Consisting of a series of statements describing the laws, theoretical principles, or beliefs, a theory summarizes and explains observations and provides a basis for making predictions about the behavior studied. By definition, theoretical principles are tentative and require further research to be deemed valid (Lefrancois, 2006). These statements or hypotheses require thorough examination through experimental observation and manipulations. Beliefs are statements that are often personal observations and are even less substantiated by experimental results than theoretical principles. Laws, on the other hand, represent statements with accuracy beyond reasonable doubt; theories in the natural sciences such as chemistry and physics are characterized by a number of laws.

Applied sciences such as physical and occupational therapy have typically relied on theoretical principles and beliefs rather than laws. Theoretical frameworks adopted in applied professions are not merely esoteric descriptions of observations and predictions; they guide clinical decision making. Theories of infant motor development provide a platform to generate hypotheses or predictions about which factors influence the emergence of gross motor skills. These hypotheses then inform assessment and intervention approaches for infants who are either at risk for motor delay or who are exhibiting motor dysfunction.

A paradigm shift in theoretical frameworks used to explain infant motor development has occurred over the last 3 decades. An array of contemporary theoretical frameworks has replaced the established neuromaturational theory (NMT) that dominated clinical approaches to gross motor assessment and intervention for young infants for almost a century. The new frameworks have been described collectively as "developmental systems" theories (Ulrich, 2010) and include specific theories such as dynamic systems theory (DST) (Thelen & Bates, 1994), neuronal group selection theory (NGST) (Sporns & Edelman, 1993), neuroconstructivism (Karmiloff-Smith, 2006),

---

[1]The term *parents* is used to represent families and caregivers of varying structures.
[2]Throughout this manual we refer to therapists; however, the Alberta Infant Motor Scale (AIMS) is appropriate for use by other health professionals who have a knowledge of infant gross motor development.

probabilistic epigenesis (Gottlieb & Lickliter, 2007), and perception action theory (Gibson, 1988). All of these theoretical frameworks reject the NMT tenet that motor skill maturation is primarily dependent on neurological maturation. Instead they present interactionist models of development that consider factors within the child, the environment, and the parameters of the functional task that behave synergistically to modulate the appearance of infant gross motor skills. Child-related influences include neurological, behavioral, and physical factors. Neurological integrity has a major impact on an infant's movement choices, but contemporary theories also consider how other child factors such as muscle strength, range of motion, anthropometric ratios, temperament, cognition, and motivation modify motor behavior. Environmental influences represent external factors not related to a specific task. For example, gravity is a significant environmental factor shaping an infant's motor abilities in the first few months after birth. Other examples of environmental factors that may influence motor maturation include noise level, ambient temperature, and even restrictive clothing. Caregivers' influence on motor development is also receiving increasing interest. A review by Spittle and Treyvaud (2016) suggest that parents and the parent-infant relationship have the strongest influence on infant development.

Gross motor skills are universally represented by descriptions of motor milestones such as rolling, reaching, sitting independently, creeping, and pulling to stand. Functional motor tasks represent the choices that infants use to explore their environments. Specific characteristics of the task can influence the functional motor solution infants use to accomplish a motor skill. For example, when first pulling to stand, depending on the height of the surface, infants may change their strategy from pulling up with their arms to using their legs. Or when creeping on a rough surface, infants may choose to creep on hands and feet (bear-walking) rather than on hands and knees. Functional motor solutions are influenced by environmental constraints and facilitators.

In this chapter we review the constructs of three theoretical frameworks. Traditional NMT is included because many of its assumptions are still evident in current therapeutic clinical decision making (Rahlin et al., 2019). DST and NGST are discussed because contemporary assessment and intervention strategies are based on these two theories (Akhbari Ziegler et al., 2019). Commonalities and differences across the three theoretical frameworks are highlighted, and the implications for assessment and therapy intervention for infants at risk of or demonstrating atypical gross motor development are discussed.

NEUROMATURATIONAL THEORY

Until the 1980s NMT theory dominated the literature describing how infant motor skills appear and mature in the neonate, infant, and toddler. Arnold Gesell (1945), Myrtle McGraw (1945), and Mary Shirley (1931) undertook meticulous longitudinal studies to document the evolution of infant motor skills over time and to link that evolution to neurological maturation. The primary tenet of their NMT framework was that the emergence of infant motor skills is dependent on the inhibition of the subcortical centers of the brain as a result of the maturation of the motor cortex. Their hypotheses were influenced by the work of neuroanatomical and embryological researchers such as Coghill (1929) and Hooker (1952) who were investigating the direct relationship between stimulation of brain structures and motor output. Their work gave rise to a neuromaturationist paradigm suggesting that neural maturation dictated infant motor behaviors.

Gesell, McGraw, and Shirley independently followed cohorts of infants from the first few weeks following birth to the emergence of independent walking and beyond, documenting not only the chronological appearance of new motor skills but also providing explanations of how they emerged. From rigorous longitudinal observation of infants, they described the emergence of motor skills according to three patterns of maturation: reflexive to voluntary, cephalocaudal, and proximal to distal. Reflex movements preceded controlled voluntary movement. Purposeful movements emerged in a predictable manner; an infant achieved head control before trunk and pelvic control, and refined hand function appeared only after proximal shoulder control was achieved. They postulated that the primary driver of these developmental sequences was the inhibition of subcortical centers of the brain as a result of the maturation of higher cortical centers. They suggested that the blueprint for the emergence and maturation of gross motor skills was predetermined or hardwired and dependent on cortical inhibition of lower brain centers. Accordingly, they hypothesized that the environment played a secondary role, if any.

Gesell (1945) and McGraw (1935) conducted longitudinal twin studies to evaluate the influence of the environment on motor skill acquisition. One twin received scheduled controlled environmental stimulation to enhance motor development while the other twin acted as a control subject. Both researchers concluded that the environment had a negligible or minimal impact on the development of an infant's gross motor skills. Shirley (1931) sent assessors to observe 25 infants in their homes weekly in their first year of life and biweekly during their second year to document the appearance and maturation of their gross motor skills. She described the emergence of motor milestones as being orderly, that the sequence of skill development was similar across infants, and that although the speed of development may vary among infants, it had no relationship to parents' stimulation.

Gesell, McGraw, and Shirley are considered the pioneers of the NMT theoretical framework and its application to infant gross motor development. A closer examination of their work reveals that all three investigators considered factors other than neurological maturation as having an influence on infant gross motor development. Although McGraw's initial purpose in her longitudinal records of infants was, in the fashion of Coghill, ". . . determining the relationship between behavior development and maturation of neural tissues, particularly those of the brain" (McGraw, 1945, p. xi), she soon realized that this goal was not achievable due to limitations of the available technology; instead she focused on documenting the maturation of motor skills. She viewed motor development as an interaction between neuroanatomical structure and physiological functions such as growth, not merely the maturation of the nervous system. McGraw's "bidirectional theory" suggested that infants and toddlers contributed to their own development by controlling how much conscious effort they made to combine alternative strategies. She also introduced the concept of "critical periods" of development, defined as a time when an infant may be most ready to explore a new motor skill.

Gesell (1945) also acknowledged the influence of physical growth on motor development. His concept of "reciprocal interweaving" suggests that some basic motor functions diverge from each other when under the influence of other traits such as growth and then recombine into a more mature motor function independent of cortical inhibition. In the same manner, Shirley (1931) kept records of children's height, weight, and head circumference and postulated that critical ratios of height and weight may influence the emergence of independent walking. While all three investigators discussed the variability of the emergence of infant motor skills, these observations were often overlooked due to their focus on documenting the average age of attainment of motor milestones. Developmental milestones became their legacy, and as a result some of the depth of their discussions has been lost. However, even though their descriptions of the emergence of infant motor skills included how internal and external factors other than cortical maturation could *influence* motor skills, they never considered how environmental factors could initiate motor solutions. Contemporary theories of motor development introduced this concept.

A SHIFT IN THEORETICAL THINKING

The advancement of neonatal intensive care for preterm infants in the 1970s stimulated renewed interest in infant gross motor development and a reevaluation of some of the assumptions of NMT. Touwen (1978) questioned the emphasis on reflex responses. He preferred using the term *reactions* rather than *reflexes* and concluded that a healthy neonate can respond to the same stimulus with a variety of motor responses. He suggested that variability in motor responses was a characteristic of typical development and that stereotypical responses in a neonate could be an indicator of abnormality. Improved ultrasound technology in the 1980s allowed real-time observations of the elegant, complex movement capabilities of a fetus. Prechtl (1984) recorded the development and continuity of fetal movements from 7.5 to 8 weeks postmenstrual age to 6 months postterm and documented in detail the quantitative and qualitative changes in neonatal motor responses. These descriptions of the maturation of fetal movements did not align with the prescriptive reflex model put forward by the NMT. At the same time alternative theoretical frameworks to explain infant motor development appeared in the literature. Two theories that have had an important influence on contemporary motor assessment and intervention approaches for young infants are the DST and NGST.

Dynamic Systems Theory

Dynamic systems principles emerged from the nonlinear dynamics of chaos theory (Gleick, 1987) described in the natural sciences literature of physics, mathematics, and biology. Researchers in these fields observed that when elements of a system work together, novel behaviors or patterns emerge that cannot be predicted from the individual contributing elements. Bernstein (1967) described a similar concept to explain adult movement by rejecting the belief that muscles were controlled individually by the central nervous system in a feedback manner. He suggested that motor choices in adults were determined by the self-organization of functional muscle synergies using information from neurological, muscular, and nonmuscular structures such as tendons and joints. He also postulated that muscle force information associated with the supporting surface could modulate the motor synergy used.

Esther Thelen, a psychologist, introduced the concepts of chaos theory and DST to the landscape of infant motor skills (Thelen et al., 1987). Her early work observing primary stepping in young infants questioned the assumption that primary stepping was a reflex integrated by cortical inhibition (Thelen et al., 1984). Her experiments revealed that the primary stepping reflex "disappeared" in infants by adding weights to their thighs and that the reflex "reappeared" in infants who no longer demonstrated the reflex when she altered the environment by holding them in a standing position in water. These findings challenged long-held beliefs about infant motor development in two important ways. First, Thelen postulated that the disappearance of primary stepping was due to a critical fat:muscle ratio in the thighs of growing infants that made the leg too heavy to continue stepping. This hypothesis contradicted the belief that neurological maturation and reflex inhibition were solely responsible for the disappearance of reflex walking, thereby suggesting that other internal mechanisms or subsystems could affect motor output. Second, she demonstrated that an external change in environment could change the motor behavior of infants.

These two ideas have become tenets of contemporary descriptions of infant motor development. Her subsequent research on infant kicking and reaching (Thelen et al., 1993) supported her beliefs that motor skills emerged as a result of self-organization of an array of parameters within the child, the task, and the environment. No single subsystem can be considered the prime causal factor for the emergence of a new motor skill. Thelen also suggested that subsystems within the child do not mature at the same rate or in a linear fashion; a small change in an important subsystem or "control parameter" can result in a new motor behavior. Conversely, any subsystem within the child, task, or environment can act as a "rate-limiting factor," impeding the emergence of a new motor skill. Infant motor solutions at any one point in time are flexible and the product of the dynamic interaction among many contributing factors within the child, the environment, and the specific task (Thelen et al., 1987). Thelen proposed that the functional task is the integral factor that shapes motor behavior. Interestingly, McGraw (1985), when reflecting on her academic research, wrote that in her twin study she had impeded the toddler's ability to ride a tricycle by strapping his feet to the pedals. She concluded that by manipulating the task instead of permitting the child to craft his own solution, she had made it more difficult for the child to perform the task. As such, she adopted a dynamic systems perspective, suggesting that the characteristics of the task shape an infant's motor solution.

Thelen continued to apply the tenets of DST to cognition (Thelen & Smith, 1994) and language (Thelen & Bates, 1994), and generated universal principles of development that could be applied across developmental domains. The first principle is the concept of nonlinear interactions of multiple internal and external subsystems influencing behaviors. The second principle is that the resultant behaviors are loosely assembled, allowing for variability of solutions over time and environments. The third principle is individuality, that children may choose different solutions for the same motor task. The fourth principle is described as embodiment, the suggestion that perception, action, and cognition are interrelated and cannot be partitioned into different developmental processes. Thelen constructed "a grand theory of dynamic systems" (Spencer et al., 2006)

to explain changes in all developmental domains. Her research has challenged occupational and physical therapists to revisit a long-held belief system grounded in NMT that has guided clinical identification and intervention principles used with neonates and infants at risk for motor dysfunction for almost a century. One of the challenges of the DST framework is that it does not identify specific neural mechanisms responsible for the initiation of motor maturation—that is, how does the spiraling, interactive process begin (Sporns & Edelman, 1993)? Neuronal group selection theory draws attention to the neurological origins of motor maturation, while incorporating the influence of the environment and task.

Neuronal Group Selection Theory

NGST has been described as a "bridge" between the NMT and DST frameworks (Hadders-Algra, 2000) because it acknowledges the influence of both nature (genetics) and nurture (environment and task) on the emergence and refinement of infant gross motor skills. Edelman (1987) proposed NGST as an overarching theory to explain how the maturational processes that occur in the brain and nervous system affect all areas of development. Sporns and Edelman (1993) applied this theory specifically to sensory motor development. Working from Bernstein's premise that movement occurs in synergies, not through individual muscle actions, they suggested that maturation of movement results from coordination among the musculoskeletal and neurological systems and afferent stimulation from the environment. Their specific interest was how changes in the brain were related to both muscle coordination and environmental influences.

NGST proposes that movement variability is a critical component of infant motor development. At birth, movement is organized through diffuse, disorganized neuronal circuits in cortical and subcortical areas of the brain. Interconnected neurons that fire in a temporally coordinated manner form neuronal groups that produce more organized movement patterns. These primary movement repertoires are not hardwired or stereotyped across all infants; their variability is a product of genetic information that provides general movement constraints for movement choices. While primary movement repertoires do not provide specific solutions to environmental situations or tasks, these movements are more organized than those at birth.

As an infant matures and practices primary movement repertoires, the brain receives increased afferent information from the environment, resulting in the emergence of secondary movement patterns linked to specific tasks and environmental situations. Although both primary and secondary movement patterns exhibit variability, the source of variability differs. Primary movement variability is a product of genetics and internal afferent information, while secondary movement patterns are a result of added external afferent information from environmental experience. These secondary movement choices are situational and task specific, appearing at different ages for different tasks.

The most mature form of secondary movement patterns evolves from one motor solution for a specific task to the emergence of multiple motor solutions for a specific motor task. This mature form of multiple solutions for one task may begin to appear for certain motor tasks as early as 2 years of age but may not appear for other more complex tasks until mature adolescence (Hadders-Algra, 2000). NGST synthesizes the interaction between neurological maturity and environmental influences; it views both as malleable and responsive. Motor maturation is not preprogrammed or hardwired; it is accomplished by initial diffuse interconnected neurons that eventually are directed to specific motor tasks as a result of afferent feedback from the environment.

The common intent of all three theories presented in this chapter is to understand and describe the process of emergence of typical infant motor skills. They differ in their explanations of the initiation of developmental changes. NMT describes inhibition of subcortical areas of the nervous system by the motor cortex as the primary instigator of change. DST views the demands of the task as the process that shapes motor behavior. NGST views diffuse epigenetic coding as the precursor of purposeful infant motor behavior. DST and NGST acknowledge that the final motor solution for any given motor task reflects an interaction of factors represented by the child, the task, and the environment. In both of these theoretical frameworks, motor development is fluid and variable, with no one preferred motor solution that may be applied across different circumstances. While McGraw and Gesell also recognized some variability in the timing and pattern of emerging motor skills both within a child and across children, their unrelenting focus on the documentation of the rate and order of the emergence of universal motor milestones rather than on individual variability resulted in their adherence to the NMT.

Movement variability, both within an infant (intraindividual) and across infants (interindividual), defines typical motor development. Historically, variability in both the pattern and age of appearance of motor milestones was considered to represent measurement error (Vereijken, 2010); it was assumed that motor skills should emerge in a smooth linear fashion. The tenets of both DST and NGST suggest that infant motor skills emerge in a nonlinear manner. Nonlinear, unique individual patterns in the development of infants' growth rates of height and weight have been reported (Lampl et al., 2001; Mei et al., 2004).

In the same manner, the appearance of infant motor skills can be episodic with many skills appearing in a short time coupled with periods of consolidation when no new motor skills emerge. Longitudinal studies of typically developing infants' scores on gross motor, fine motor, and language developmental scales have revealed variability both in an individual infant's score over time and among infants' scores at one time (Darrah et al., 1998, 2003). Infants do not maintain the same percentile score at all sampling ages, and there is not one universal pattern of the emergence of infant motor skills. Previous studies of emerging motor milestones may have failed to capture these patterns of intraindividual and interindividual variability because the time interval between assessments in most longitudinal studies of infant development is long and thus may fail to capture the discontinuous shape of development (Adolph et al., 2008). Factors that affect variability can be intrinsic to the infant such as anthropometric change (height, weight, strength), behavioral characteristics (temperament, curiosity), and cognitive abilities. External factors associated with the environment or the demands of the task can also affect an infant's movement solution. For example, an infant with a mature gait may revert to a high guard pattern when walking on uneven surfaces, or an infant may creep to move in her home but decides to bear-walk on hands and knees when outside on an unfamiliar surface.

In summary, contemporary theories of infant motor development reject the premise that motor skills are hardwired and dependent solely on cortical maturation. In addition to neurological integrity, many other physiologic and behavioral characteristics within an infant can influence motor behavior. Characteristics of the task and the environment also contribute to an infant's motor solutions. How have these new principles and beliefs changed the assessment and intervention approaches of therapists?

CHANGING THEORIES, CHANGING PRACTICE

NMT dominated the landscape of infant motor development for over 50 years; as such, the theory informed and defined infant motor assessments and intervention principles during this time. Approaches to assessment were prescriptive and followed a reflex to voluntary movement pattern. Accordingly, therapists evaluated the integration of primitive reflexes, the emergence of righting and equilibrium reactions, and changes in muscle tone and resting postures, with little or no consideration of environmental influences. This assessment approach required extensive handling of the infant by the therapist, who often placed the infant in unnatural positions such as vertical and ventral suspension. Infants were expected to follow a similar course of motor development both in terms of the sequence of appearance of motor skills and the rate of appearance. Interindividual or intraindividual variability in patterns of movement were viewed as error or "noise" rather than an integral feature of emerging motor skills.

Traditional intervention programs for infants with motor disorders also were based on the assumptions underlying NMT. Extensive handling of an infant by the therapist attempted to inhibit "abnormal" patterns of movement and to facilitate "normal" patterns of movement. Treatment approaches included suppressing primitive reflexes, encouraging head control before trunk control, developing proximal shoulder control before voluntary hand control, and practicing sitting and four-point kneeling before standing. An infant's movement was controlled by the therapist, and the therapist determined the optimal movement solution for an activity. For example, infants with increased muscle tone who were able to pull to stand using bilateral hip and knee extension may have been discouraged from standing until they could master a more "mature" dissociated pattern of movement through half-kneeling.

Interactionist theories such as DST and NGST have modified therapists' perspectives of assessment and intervention approaches for infants at risk for motor delay and those with identified motor dysfunction. The tenets of these theories encourage therapists to consider the spontaneous motor solutions of infants as innovative rather than abnormal. Infant assessment tools have evolved from therapist-initiated testing of primitive reflexes, righting reactions, and equilibrium reactions to more hands-off approaches that entail observing the spontaneous movements of infants. The quality and variability of infant movements are considered important indicators of typical motor maturation. Motor milestones continue to provide a window into an infant's motor progress but with the understanding that they represent the outcome of development, not the process of development (Adolph et al., 2008).

Intervention approaches based on DST and NGST frameworks are now occurring in clinical practice (Akhbari Ziegler et al., 2019; Law et al., 2007; Löwing et al., 2009; Morgan et al., 2016). These approaches focus on the achievement of child- and parent-identified functional goals rather than therapist-identified goals. The interventions are multifaceted and consider an array of factors within the child, the task, and the environment that may act as either barriers or facilitators to the achievement of the identified goal. There is an appreciation for child-initiated exploration of movement. Opportunities for practice are important; innovative movement solutions and environmental modifications are valued. Therapists no longer assume that there is one "best" motor solution that applies to all infants; rather they may provide opportunities for an infant to explore a variety of motor solutions to achieve the same functional task.

Similarly, traditional models of intervention are not supported using DST or NGST principles. The following clinical example highlights some of the assessment and intervention differences based on the NMT and contemporary theoretical models.

> Amy is 8 months old with a diagnosis of mild spastic hemiplegia on her right side. She is curious and enjoys exploring her environment by rolling. She can maintain sitting when placed in the position. She recently learned a new way to move in sitting by "scooting" on her buttocks (bottom shuffling). Her parents are very proud that she has learned this new skill and want to share her achievement with her therapist.

Using the concepts of NMT, therapists might advise the parents to discourage "bottom shuffling" because of concern that it would promote further asymmetry. To achieve more symmetric motor behavior they might place Amy in a four-point kneeling position and encourage creeping to replace bottom shuffling. In contrast, using the concept of DST or NGST, therapists would respect, even celebrate, Amy's new motor skill achievement with her parents and let Amy continue practicing her new skill. They also might ensure that Amy had opportunities to experience movement symmetry by modifying her environment and her motor tasks. For example, they might suggest toys that encourage the use of both hands and suggest that the parents place toys on a higher surface so that Amy can experience symmetry in standing. They would encourage opportunities for Amy to explore a variety of movement strategies but would not restrict Amy's spontaneous movement solutions.

Therapy approaches derived from DST and NGST are not congruent with treatment principles based on tenets of the NMT. Even though DST and NGST frameworks are prevalent in the literature and are taught in entry-level professional programs, clinical interventions continue to incorporate many NMT-derived practices such as infant movement that is controlled by the therapist, preferred movement solutions, and the assumption that motor control should follow a cephalocaudal, proximal-to-distal sequence. A disconnect between contemporary theoretical frameworks and clinical decision making and interventions is still present (Rahlin et al., 2019).

FUTURE CHALLENGES

McGraw (1985) wrote an essay confessing six personal "blunders" of her career. Her fifth blunder was labeled "Theories." She reflected:

Over the years colleagues have commented that I never attempted to formulate a McGraw Theory of early behavior development. . . . An explanation for my failure to do so is quite simple. At the time I was not qualified with an understanding of the artistry and techniques of theory formation, nor did I have the mathematical skill to do so. Perhaps therein lies my blunder. My concept was of multisystems developmental processes emerging and advancing at different times and different rates, but finally interacting, integrating and synthesizing for the creation of new performances or traits. I preferred to present my findings as observed and to allow future researchers to make use of them as they saw fit. Had I attempted to formulate a theory for such a complex of processes then decorated it with a catchy acronym, the chances are that it would soon have been challenged by some current or future investigator and then we would have another troublesome dichotomy to deal with. . . . Perhaps some future or present-day investigator can formulate a comprehensive theory of development that can withstand dichotomies. The subtle complex processes deserve a reliable, workable theory. (p. 170)

Perhaps if McGraw had ventured to develop a theoretical framework from her observations, it would have resembled the concepts of DST and NGST. Contemporary interactionist theorists suggest, as McGraw did, that development is an interactive, integrated, and synthesized process characterized by variability rather than uniformity. Has her vision of a reliable, workable theory been reached? At present the process of infant motor development is not explained by one universally accepted theory. Tenets of different theories overlap, making it confusing to disentangle the terminology and specific premises of each theory. Unfortunately, the efficacy of the emerging therapeutic programs based on these theories has not yet been confirmed (Morgan et al., 2016). More research is needed to evaluate whether the theories can, indeed, be supported by clinical interventions based on a unified therapy approach.

Perhaps one unified therapy approach to the assessment and intervention of infants at risk for motor disorders is not reasonable considering the complexity of infant motor maturation and the new understanding of the variability in motor solutions. Instead a "menu" of clinical assessment and intervention options based on theory and research may better guide therapists in making informed clinical choices tailored to the characteristics of an individual infant and a specific functional goal. There may be an array of intervention solutions to achieve a functional goal with the most effective solution differing for each infant. Such diversity of both individual motor solutions and therapy approaches makes evaluation of the effectiveness of interventions more challenging. New research evaluation methods may also need to be developed, as the gold standard randomized controlled trial may not prove to be the best method to use when evaluating the efficacy of new intervention approaches.

Infant motor development theory has evolved from prescriptive brain-controlled beliefs to contemporary frameworks that consider the role of numerous interacting variables within the infant, the task, and the environment that shape an infant's motor solution. Contemporary theories of infant motor control have made the understanding of infant motor development more complex and hence more challenging to translate easily into practice. The challenge for physical and occupational therapists is to avoid repeating the error of blindly accepting the new theories, as was done with NMT, as truth. Theories are not truth; rather they are a set of assumptions to describe observations and as such need to be systematically evaluated. Occupational and physical therapists are well positioned, using innovative research methods, to evaluate assessment and intervention protocols based on the new theoretical paradigms, thereby linking practice to the underlying theory.

REFERENCES

Adolph, K. E., Robinson, S. R., Young, J. W., & Gill-Alvarez, F. (2008). What is the shape of developmental change? *Psychological Review, 115*(3), 527–543.

Akhbari Ziegler, S., Dirks, T., & Hadders-Algra, M. (2019). Coaching in early physical therapy intervention: The COPCA program as an example of translation of theory into practice. *Disability and Rehabilitation, 41*(15), 1846–1854.

Bernstein, N. (1967). *The coordination and regulation of movement.* Pergamon.

Coghill, G. (1929). *Anatomy and the problem of behavior.* Cambridge University Press.

Darrah, J., Hodge, M., Magill-Evans, J., & Kembhavi, G. (2003). Stability of serial assessments of motor and communication abilities in typically developing infants—implications for screening. *Early Human Development, 72*(2), 97–110.

Darrah, J., Redfern, L., Maguire, T. O., Beaulne, A. P., & Watt, J. (1998). Intra-individual stability of rate of gross motor development in full-term infants. *Early Human Development, 52*(2), 169–179.

Edelman, G. M. (1987). *Neural Darwinism: The theory of neuronal group selection.* Basic Books.

Gesell, A. (1945). *The embryology of behavior, the beginnings of the human mind.* Harper and Brothers.

Gibson, E. J. (1988). Exploratory behavior in the development of perceiving, acting, and the acquiring of knowledge. *Annual Review of Psychology, 39*, 1–41.

Gleick, J. (1987). *Chaos: Making a new science.* Penguin.

Gottlieb, G., & Lickliter, R. (2007). Probabilistic epigenesis. *Developmental Science, 10*(1), 1–11.

Hadders-Algra, M. (2000). The neuronal group selection theory: Promising principles for understanding and treating developmental motor disorders. *Developmental Medicine and Child Neurology, 42*(10), 707–715.

Hooker, D. (1952). *The prenatal origin of behavior.* University of Kansas Press.

Karmiloff-Smith, A. (2006). The tortuous route from genes to behavior: A neuroconstructivist approach. *Cognitive, Affective and Behavioral Neuroscience, 6*(1), 9–17.

Lampl, M., Johnson, M. L., & Frongillo, E. A. (2001). Mixed distribution analysis identifies saltation and stasis growth. *Annals of Human Biology, 28*(4), 403–411.

Law, M., Darrah, J., Pollock, N., Rosenbaum, P., Russell, D., Walter, S. D., Petrenchik, T., Wilson, B., & Wright, V. (2007). Focus on function—a randomized controlled trial comparing two rehabilitation interventions for young children with cerebral palsy. *BMC Pediatrics, 7.*

Lefrancois, G. R. (2006). *Theories of human learning* (5th ed.). Thomson Wadsworth.

Löwing, K., Bexelius, A., & Brogren Carlberg, E. (2009). Activity focused and goal directed therapy for children with cerebral palsy—do goals make a difference? *Disability and Rehabilitation, 31*(22), 1808–1816.

McGraw, M. B. (1935). *Growth: A study of Johnny and Jimmy.* Appleton-Century-Crofts.

McGraw, M. B. (1945). *The neuromuscular maturation of the human infant* (Reprint ed.). Hafner Publishing Company.

McGraw, M. B. (1985). Professional and personal blunders in child development research. *The Psychological Record, 35*(2), 165–170.

Mei, Z., Grummer-Strawn, L. M., Thompson, D., & Dietz, W. H. (2004). Shifts in percentiles of growth during early childhood: Analysis of longitudinal data from the California Child Health and Development Study. *Pediatrics, 113*(6), 617–627.

Morgan, C., Darrah, J., Gordon, A. M., Harbourne, R., Spittle, A., Johnson, R., & Fetters, L. (2016). Effectiveness of motor interventions in infants with cerebral palsy: A systematic review. *Developmental Medicine and Child Neurology, 58*(9), 900–909.

Prechtl, H. F. R. (1984). Continuity of neural functions from prenatal to postnatal life. *Clinics in Developmental Medicine, 94,* 1–15.

Rahlin, M., Barnett, J., Becker, E., & Fregosi, C. M. (2019). Development through the lens of a perception-action-cognition connection: Recognizing the need for a paradigm shift in clinical reasoning. *Physical Therapy, 99*(6), 748–760.

Shirley, M. (1931). *The first two years: A study of twenty-five babies.* University of Minnesota Press.

Spencer, J. P., Clearfield, M., Corbetta, D., Ulrich, B., Buchanan, P., & Schöner, G. (2006). Moving toward a grand theory in development: In memory of Esther Thelen. *Child Development, 77*(6), 1521–1538.

Spittle, A., & Treyvaud, K. (2016). The role of early developmental intervention to influence neurobehavioral outcomes of children born preterm. *Seminars in Perinatology, 40*(8), 542–548.

Sporns, O., & Edelman, G. M. (1993). Solving Bernstein's problem: A proposal for the development of coordinated movement by selection. *Child Development, 64*(4), 960–981.

Thelen, E., & Bates, L. B. (1994). *A dynamic systems approach to the development of cognition and action.* MIT Press.

Thelen, E., Corbetta, D., Kamm, K., Spencer, J. P., Schneider, K., & Zernicke, R. F. (1993). The transition to reaching: Mapping intention and intrinsic dynamics. *Child Development, 64*(4), 1058–1098.

Thelen, E., Fisher, D. M., & Ridley-Johnson, R. (1984). The relationship between physical growth and a newborn reflex. *Infant Behavior and Development, 7*(4), 479–493.

Thelen, E., Kelso, J. A. S., & Fogel, A. (1987). Self-organizing systems and infant motor development. *Developmental Review, 7*(1), 39–65.

Thelen, E., & Smith, L. B. (1994). *A dynamic systems approach to the development of cognition and action.* MIT Press.

Touwen, B. C. L. (1978). Variability and stereotypy in normal and deviant development. In J. Apply (Ed.), *Care of the handicapped child. Clinics in developmental medicine* (No. 67, pp. 99–110). JB Lippincott.

Ulrich, B. D. (2010). Opportunities for early intervention based on theory, basic neuroscience, and clinical science. *Physical Therapy, 90*(12), 1868–1880.

Vereijken, B. (2010). The complexity of childhood development: Variability in perspective. *Physical Therapy, 90*(12), 1850–1859.

2

Motor Assessment of the Developing Infant

Alicia Spittle

BACKGROUND

Motor assessments, also known as measurement tools, are a fundamental component of health professionals tool kit, such as physical therapy and occupational therapy. An assessment process includes both a subjective assessment, gathering information regarding the purpose for the assessment and the clinical history, and an objective assessment, which may include a standardized motor assessment. A standardized measure provides a systematic method to administer and to score an assessment, allowing therapists to compare results with each other or with themselves the next time they conduct an assessment. Standardized assessments are usually norm referenced, where the performance of an individual is compared with a specific population, while criterion referenced is where an individual has to meet specific criteria and the performance is contrasted with the test content rather than a population (Spittle et al., 2008).

Pediatric therapists complete infant motor assessments for different reasons and with different populations of children. Developmental surveillance of preterm infants at high risk for motor impairments because of their birth history includes ongoing motor assessments at different ages; most of these infants will not have permanent motor delays or impairments. For infants with a definite diagnosis early in life, serial motor assessments are an important component of their ongoing management; the assessments provide a record of an infant's motor progress and may capture the effects of intervention. Therapists also assess infants who have no adverse birth history but whose parents or caregivers are concerned that their infant is delayed; a motor assessment may be used to compare their infant's development with test norms (Orton et al., 2018; Rosenbaum, 1998).

The unique characteristics of infant motor maturation make standardized objective assessments challenging.

Infant motor skills evolve over time and for typically developing infants the rate of change may be rapid and variable (Adolph & Franchak, 2017). The emergence of motor skills in the first year of life is not a linear process, and a consistent or predictable change in scores over serial assessments cannot be expected. The rationale for why a motor assessment is required may also change over time. Initially, it could be to identify if an infant has delayed development, but as the infant gets older the therapist may want to evaluate the infant's response to intervention over time.

These various characteristics of infant motor maturation make the choice of the appropriate assessment measure challenging. Because there are numerous infant motor measures to choose from, it can be confusing to decide on the best measure to use for each infant. It is essential that therapists understand their reason for choosing a particular motor assessment tool and how effective the standardized assessment tool will be to achieve the desired purpose. This chapter discusses how infant assessments differ from the assessment processes used with older children, continues with the important role of parents in infant assessments, and concludes with an overview of the psychometric properties and purposes of standardized measures.

INFANT ASSESSMENTS—THE UNIQUE CHALLENGES

Infant motor assessments are inherently more challenging than the assessment procedures used with older children. When working with older children, a diagnosis has usually already been established, and the assessor is evaluating factors associated with the diagnosis that are either limiting or enhancing motor performance. In contrast, when assessing infants, it is often uncertain whether the infant's motor performance represents a short-term developmental delay or a long-term motor impairment. Most infants who are assessed will not have yet received a diagnosis, and many of these infants will go on to have typical gross motor development. Thus the assessor needs to understand both the components of movement that are observed in typical motor development and the motor strategies that represent or signal deviations from typical development.

Unlike older children, infants are unable to voluntarily demonstrate what they can and cannot do or why they are having challenges with movement. An infant assessment requires that the assessor observe the infant moving spontaneously rather than working cooperatively with the child to elicit specific movements. There may be numerous explanations for why an infant may be having difficulty with a particular motor skill. For example, if a 9-month-old infant is unable to sit independently, the assessor needs to determine the factors that may be contributing to the delay: is it because of hypertonia, hypotonia, contractures, poor righting reactions, illness, shyness, cognitive delay, or perhaps the fact that the infant has had very little experience in the position? The assessor has to consider all the factors that may contribute to a motor delay and systematically rule them out.

While all pediatric assessments should be fun and play based, this is particularly important for infants as they may be nonverbal, unable to understand verbal instructions, easily distracted, or tire easily (LoBue et al., 2020).

WORKING WITH PARENTS AND CAREGIVERS

Parents and/or caregivers should to be engaged with and actively participate in their infant's assessment. It is important that they understand the purpose of the assessment (including what the assessment can and cannot do), actively participate in the administration of the test measure (where appropriate), and be fully informed of the results of the assessment. Generally, infants are more secure when a familiar face is present. Parents know their infant best and are able to guide the assessor regarding their infant's current interests and skill level. For example, the parent may share that their infant likes to sit, thereby cueing the assessor that sitting may be a good position for starting the assessment. Some assessment tools require that the test is conducted in a standardized order; even then, parents may be present for the assessment and assist in pacing the assessment with breaks for soothing if the infant becomes upset. Assessment results need to be communicated sensitively with parents, and they may need assistance to interpret a test score and its implications. It is extremely important that the infant's strengths are highlighted as well as any identified concerns (Novak et al., 2017).

WHAT ARE THE IMPORTANT PSYCHOMETRIC PROPERTIES OF AN ASSESSMENT TOOL?

Infant assessments are complex with unique challenges, but like all standardized measurement tools they need to have strong psychometric properties, including reliability, responsiveness, and validity (Mokkink et al., 2010). The reliability of an assessment tool is comprised of three measurement properties: internal consistency (the degree of interrelatedness among items), reliability (the degree of measurement stability between different assessors [interrater], the same assessor on a different occasion [intrarater], or over time [test-retest]), and measurement error (the systematic and random error that is not attributed to true change in the construct being measured). A certain amount of measurement error or noise is always present. The challenge of infant assessments is to validly determine the amount of change that is clinically meaningful. Interpreting change in an infant's score over time or even between assessors at the same time is particularly challenging due to the variability of typical motor development (Darrah et al., 1998b; Spittle et al., 2008).

Responsiveness refers to the ability of an assessment to detect change over time related to the construct being measured. Responsiveness is considered its own measurement property according to Consensus-based Standards for the Selection of Health Measurement Instruments (COSMIN) (Mokkink et al., 2010), highlighting the clinical importance of change scores. For infant assessment tools that aim to assess the effect of intervention, the measure needs to detect changes in performance that are deemed clinically important (Spittle, et al., 2008).

Validity refers to the degree to which the assessment tool measures the construct of interest and encompasses three measurement properties: content, construct, and criterion validity. Content validity is one of the most important measurement properties of an outcome measure but also the most challenging to assess (Terwee et al., 2018). Three aspects of content validity important to consider are relevance (all items should be relevant for the construct of interest within a specific population and context of use), comprehensiveness (no key aspects of the construct should be missing), and comprehensibility (the items should be understood and meaningful by the population of interest). Essential to being able to assess content validity is to identify the construct of interest of the measurement tool (i.e., the theoretical and conceptual frameworks underpinning the assessment measure). Assessments of infant motor development do not measure all motor behaviors, rather they focus on the aspects of motor development described by the underlying framework/model (Adolph & Franchak, 2017). For example, infant motor assessments based on traditional neuromaturation theories of development assess motor development as a hierarchic process, while assessment tools using contemporary theories of motor development such as the dynamic systems theory consider the influence of the environment and how the infant interacts with the environment. These assessments consider the infant in a more active role (e.g., Does the infant reach for a toy?) rather than observing how the infant responds to a stimulus (e.g., reflex testing). Criterion validity refers to the degree in which an assessment is an adequate reflection of a gold standard assessment. This could include how well sequential scores on different assessment measures correlate with each other, such as the Alberta Infant Motor Scale (AIMS) and Bayley standard scores. Alternatively, it could assess how well an assessment classifies an infant's development compared to a gold standard classification; an example would be the comparison of the AIMS centile rank below a certain cutoff score and a pediatrician's assessment of normal versus suspicious/delayed development (Darrah et al., 1998a; Spittle et al., 2008).

PURPOSE OF THE MOTOR ASSESSMENT

The availability of so many infant motor assessments challenges therapists to determine which measure to use and when. Kirchner and Guyatt (1985) described a methodological framework to assess health status that has been widely adopted and is still referenced in discussions of health measures. Their framework suggests that health measures are developed to be used for one or more of three purposes: discrimination, prediction, and evaluation (as mentioned earlier).

A discriminative tool distinguishes between individuals on a particular dimension or characteristic. The discrimination is based on an infant's current performance compared to a reference group. Norm-referenced measures serve this purpose; they categorize children by means of percentile rank scores, standard scores, or age-equivalent scores. Examples of such indices include the Bayley Scales of Infant and Toddler Development (Bayley & Alyward, 2019) and the Peabody Developmental Motor Scales, 2nd edition (Folio & Fewell, 2000). Scales like these are intended to identify children who are demonstrating below average performance when compared to infants in the reference or normative group. These instruments are usually standardized on large populations to ensure acceptable reliability and validity. When using discriminative assessments, it is important to take into consideration where (e.g., country, culture), with whom (e.g., low-risk, at-risk, and high-risk infants), and when (e.g., year) the normative data were collected and their appropriateness when applied to the population at hand. For example, the Bayley

3rd edition normative data (Bayley, 2006) were from the United States and included children who are typically developing and with developmental disabilities, and when used with Australian children born preterm, it was found to underestimate motor impairments because of cultural, social, and environmental differences between the countries (Spittle et al., 2013).

The prediction of future performance is the purpose of a predictive tool that classifies individuals into categories based on what is expected to be their future status. Predictive tools often classify children into two categories, such as "normal vs abnormal" or "subsicious/sub-optimal"; with young infants there may be a third "suspicious" category. An example of a predictive assessment tool for infants is the Prechtl General Movement Assessment (GMA) (Einspieler et al., 2005), which may be used to predict an individual infant's risk of developmental impairment, including cerebral palsy. The important psychometric properties of predictive indices are sensitivity (i.e., the ability for a test to detect someone with a condition, such as cerebral palsy), specificity (i.e., the ability for the test to detect someone without a condition, such as not having cerebral palsy), positive predictive value (i.e., the probability that someone with a positive test will have a condition), and negative predictive value (i.e., the probability that someone with a negative test truly does not have the condition). Few tests attain 100% sensitivity, specificity, and positive and negative predictive values; rather it is matter of balancing an acceptable level of sensitivity/positive predictive value with an acceptable level of specificity/negative predictive values so that infants with a condition are detected and infants without the condition are not falsely identified as having the condition. Because the predictive validity of a test is influenced by not only the prevalence of the condition but also by biological, environment, cultural, and social factors, predicting an individual infant's later outcome is challenging (Adolph & Franchak, 2017; Spittle et al., 2008).

Differences in caregiving practices and the way an infant interacts with the environment may influence both the timing of skill development and the shape of an infant's developmental trajectory. For this reason, it is recommended that a combination of assessments be employed, including repeat assessments over time, neurological assessments, and neuroimaging (when available) coupled with clinical histories, to predict an infant's outcome and ultimate diagnosis. Although we need to consider psychometric properties related to diagnostic accuracy of a test, such as sensitivity and specificity, there are currently no infant motor assessments with predictive validity for use solely as a diagnostic tool. Rather, they form a component of the clinical picture. For example, international guidelines for early detection and diagnosis of cerebral palsy recommend combining assessment findings from a standardized motor assessment (e.g., GMA, AIMS), neurological examination (e.g., Hammersmith Infant Neurological Examination), neuroimaging (e.g., magnetic resonance imaging), and clinical history (Novak et al., 2017).

An evaluative tool is used to measure the magnitude of change in performance over time or following treatment. Such a measure should be responsive to small increments of change in motor performance, resulting from either maturation or intervention. Evaluative measures are often criterion referenced, rather than norm referenced, meaning the child may be assessed on the same or similar items over time, which enables change in the child's motor skills to be assessed (Rosenbaum, 1998). The Gross Motor Function Measure (Russell et al., 2000) is an example of an evaluative measure. It is intended to measure change in the gross motor abilities of children with cerebral palsy and was designed specifically to measure the outcome of physical therapy for children with cerebral palsy. Responsiveness is a challenging property to measure in the gross motor development of young infants. Although most infants' motor skills improve with age, theoretical concepts suggest that the maturation of motor skills is nonlinear, characterized by variability in the appearance of motor skills (Vereijken, 2010). Research suggests that typically developing infants do not maintain the same percentile ranking on standardized testing over time (Darrah et al., 1998b). Variability and nonlinearity of infant motor skills characterize typical infant motor development and make it challenging to assess change over time in response to therapy and beyond what is expected from maturation. When choosing an evaluative tool, it is important to know the characteristics of the evaluated population and whether it is appropriate to use with other populations. For example, when assessing change over time in children with cerebral palsy, it is important that the tool has been validated in this population. If an assessment tool shown to be responsive with typically developing children is used with infants with cerebral palsy, it is unlikely to detect clinically meaningful changes with these infants.

USING STANDARDIZED MOTOR ASSESSMENTS IN CLINICAL PRACTICE

It is imperative to understand the psychometric properties of any assessment tool, but it is also important to consider how feasible it is to use the tool in a specific clinical setting or practice. Factors to consider include the cost to train or purchase the assessment, the amount of time it takes to administer and score, and the training required to meet acceptable reliability standards. A motor assessment may show good interrater and intrarater reliability when performed by experts or people trained in the assessment, but it is important to know if it is reliable when used by novice clinicians or appropriate for use without training.

CONCLUSION

Infant motor assessments are complex and challenging, weaving together a variety of qualities, purposes, and skill levels. Therapists who assess infants' gross motor skills require a knowledge of both theoretical frameworks of gross motor maturation and the uses and psychometric properties of measurement tools. They need to systematically consider and evaluate the multiple factors that may influence an infant's motor solution. They need to understand that infant motor maturation is not a linear process but instead is characterized by individual variability and stability. They need to be comfortable with uncertainty, sometimes having to wait to see if their prognosis was correct. But the rewards of assessing infants' motor skills are worth the challenges. Using their knowledge to problem solve why an infant is having difficulty mastering a motor skill and how the infant's movement and/or the environment can be changed to achieve success, therapists witness the joy of an infant mastering a new motor skill and share in the parents' delight. Indeed, the infants are the instructors and the therapists, the students.

REFERENCES

Adolph, K. E., & Franchak, J. M. (2017). The development of motor behavior. *Wiley Interdisciplinary Reviews: Cognitive Science, 8*(1-2).

Bayley, N. (2006). *Bayley scales of infant and toddler development: Administration manual* (3rd ed.). Psychorp.

Bayley, N., & Alyward, G. P. (2019). *Bayley scales of infant and toddler development (Bayley-4)* (4th ed.). Pearson.

Darrah, J., Piper, M., & Watt, M. J. (1998a). Assessment of gross motor skills of at-risk infants: Predictive validity of the Alberta Infant Motor Scale. *Developmental Medicine and Child Neurology, 40*(7), 485–491.

Darrah, J., Redfern, L., Maguire, T. O., Beaulne, A. P., & Watt, J. (1998b). Intra-individual stability of rate of gross motor development in full-term infants. *Early Human Development, 52*(2), 169–179.

Einspieler, C., Prechtl, H., Bos, A. F., Ferrari, F., & Cioni, G. (2005). *Prechtl's method on the qualitative assessment of general movements in preterm, term and young infants* (Vol. 167). Cambridge University Press.

Folio, M., & Fewell, R. F. (2000). *Peabody developmental motor scales* (2nd ed.). Pro Ed.

Kirshner, B., & Guyatt, G. (1985). A methodological framework for assessing health indices. *Journal of Chronic Diseases, 38*(1), 27–36.

LoBue, V., Reider, L. B., Kim, E., Burris, J. L., Oleas, D. S., Buss, K. A., Pérez-Edgar, K., & Field, A. (2020). The importance of using multiple outcome measures in infant research. *Infancy, 25*(4), 420–437.

Mokkink, L. B., Terwee, C. B., Patrick, D. L., Alonso, J., Stratford, P. W., Knol, D. L., Bouter, L. M., & de Vet, H. C. (2010). The COSMIN study reached international consensus on taxonomy, terminology, and definitions of measurement properties for health-related patient-reported outcomes. *Journal of Clinical Epidemiology, 63*(7), 737–745.

Novak, I., Morgan, C., Adde, L., Blackman, J., Boyd, R. N., Brunstrom-Hernandez, J., Cioni, G., Damiano, D., Darrah, J., Eliasson, A., de Vries, L. S., Einspieler, C., Fahey, M., Fehlings, D., Rerriero, D. M., Fetters, L., Fiori, S., Forssberg, H., Gordon, A. M., . . . & Badawi, N. (2017). Early, accurate diagnosis and early intervention in cerebral palsy: Advances in diagnosis and treatment. *JAMA Pediatrics, 171*(9), 897–907.

Orton, J. L., Olsen, J. E., Ong, K., Lester, R., & Spittle, A. J. (2018). NICU graduates: The role of the allied health team in follow-up. *Pediatric Annals, 47*(4), e165–e171.

Rosenbaum, P. (1998). Screening tests and standardized assessments used to identify and characterize developmental delays. *Seminars in Pediatric Neurology, 5*(1), 27–32.

Russell, D. J., Avery, L. M., Rosenbaum, P. L., Raina, P. S., Walter, S. D., & Palisano, R. J. (2000). Improved scaling of the gross motor function measure for children with cerebral palsy: Evidence of reliability and validity. *Physical Therapy, 80*(9), 873–885.

Spittle, A. J., Doyle, L. W., & Boyd, R. N. (2008). A systematic review of the clinimetric properties of neuromotor assessments for preterm infants during the first year of life. *Developmental Medicine and Child Neurology, 50*(4), 254–266.

Spittle, A. J., Spencer-Smith, M. M., Eeles, A. L., Lee, K. J., Lorefice, L. E., Anderson, P. J., & Doyle, L. W. (2013). Does the Bayley-III motor scale at 2 years predict motor outcome at 4 years in very preterm children? *Developmental Medicine and Child Neurology, 55*(5), 448–452.

Terwee, C. B., Prinsen, C. A. C., Chiarotto, A., Westerman, M. J., Patrick, D. L., Alonso, J., Bouter, L. M., de Vet., H. C W., & Mokkink, L. B. (2018). COSMIN methodology for evaluating the content validity of patient-reported outcome measures: A Delphi study. *Quality of Life Research, 27*(5), 1159–1170.

Vereijken, B. (2010). The complexity of childhood development: Variability in perspective. *Physical Therapy, 90*(12), 1850–1859.

3

Alberta Infant Motor Scale: Construction of a Motor Assessment Tool for the Developing Infant

BACKGROUND

Developmental screening to detect early developmental delays in infants and young children is an important component of pediatric health care (Khan, 2019). In 2001 the American Academy of Pediatrics (AAP) recommended that all children receive developmental screening (AAP, 2001), and in 2006 the organization published an algorithm for developmental assessment that included risk assessments, developmental surveillance, screening, and diagnosis (Council on Children With Disabilities, 2006). These guidelines recommended developmental screening for all children at ages 9, 18, and 30 months using a valid, standardized psychometrically sound screening tool that covers several developmental domains. Publication of these guidelines resulted in a heightened interest in the clinical use of standardized measures for screening (Radecki et al., 2011). Universal developmental screening tests usually cover a variety of areas of development and often involve checklists that do not describe in detail the components of gross motor skills that are acknowledged as the first indicators of a delay. Because of the importance of assessing an infant's gross motor development early in the first year of life, pediatric occupational therapists and physical therapists are involved in assessing those infants who are at increased risk for gross motor delays. These professionals require gross motor measures that provide more detailed descriptions than developmental screening tests.

In 1994 when the Alberta Infant Motor Scale (AIMS) was published, improvements in neonatal intensive care units (NICUs) had resulted in an increased survival rate of preterm infants (Fanaroff et al., 2003) who are known to be at increased risk of development delays when compared with their full-term counterparts. Pediatric physical therapists and occupational therapists were members of health care teams working in neonatal follow-up clinics to identify infants with developmental challenges. Neonatal follow-up clinics continue to play an important role in monitoring the development of cohorts of NICU graduates to identify those infants who are at increased risk for neurodevelopmental impairments. Current data suggest that survival rates have increased for preterm infants born at less than 33 weeks of gestation (Lee et al., 2020); as a result, therapists are involved in assessing the gross motor development of increased numbers of at-risk infants and providing appropriate intervention if necessary.

The AIMS was developed in response to the need for a norm-referenced, psychometrically sound measure of infant gross motor development from birth to independent walking that evaluated components of gross motor maturation important to pediatric therapists and other professionals who assess at-risk infants. At the time the AIMS was constructed, the majority of standardized gross motor measures used by pediatric therapists were developed by physicians, psychologists, and educators. Measures such as the Peabody Developmental Motor Scales (Folio & Fewell, 1983) and the Bayley Scales of Infant Development (Bayley, 1969) were used for the assessment and longitudinal follow-up of at-risk infants. These measures, although psychometrically sound, were largely item or milestone based with little or no evaluation of the qualitative aspects associated with accomplishing the specific item. For example, one item on these earlier scales might be "infant rolls over" with no description of the motor components used by an infant to roll over. These earlier scales did not evaluate the specific components of gross motor skills known to be important to pediatric therapists such as an infant's weight-bearing position, rotation of trunk, and/or spontaneous active movements. Evaluation of components of movement provides important information regarding the quality of established or emerging gross motor milestones. Because of the lack of detailed descriptors of motor skills in the available assessment measures, therapists often did not use these standardized measures. Instead, there was a proliferation of in-house measures developed by individual neonatal follow-up clinics and infant neuromotor assessment programs. These measures were most often descriptive narrative reports with no standardization of testing procedures, no normative data, and no evaluation of psychometric properties such as reliability and validity.

The landscape of infant gross motor measures has changed significantly since then. An array of infant assessment tools now is available to document the emergence of infant gross motor skills. At least 18 published measures are available to use with infants 0 to 3 years of age (Effgen & Howman, 2013). The specific types of published infant measures have been classified into four categories: (1) descriptive neurological examination, (2) standardized scoring of neurological examination with or without motor behaviors, (3) observation of milestones and specific patterns of motor behavior, and (4) quality of motor behavior (Heineman & Hadders-Algra, 2008). The majority of the measures report psychometric properties and describe standardized assessment procedures. Many of the measures reflect the tenets of current theoretical frameworks of neuromotor development. Some measures require specific training of therapists to administer the measure, and some measures have constrained age ranges for use. The publication of pediatric developmental screening guidelines, the continued follow-up of at-risk infants, and the development of new infant measures have all influenced therapy practice. The use of standardized, psychometrically sound motor assessment tools is now recognized as an essential component of infant fine motor and gross motor assessments.

The AIMS was developed as a discriminative and evaluative tool. Its discriminative purpose is to identify infants who exhibited immature or delayed gross motor development compared to a large normative sample. The evaluative purpose is to document small increments in performance over time, due to either maturation or the effect of intervention. The predictive validity of the AIMS was investigated after publication of the measure and is presented in Chapter 10. The clinical uses of the AIMS are discussed in Chapter 9.

The AIMS assesses the maturation of infant gross motor skills from term (40 weeks postconception) to 18 months of age. An infant's movement choices are observed in four developmental positions; prone, supine, sit and stand. The AIMS was designed as an observational measure with minimal handling by the examiner, thereby allowing the infant to move freely without the assistance or interference of the examiner. This observational feature distinguished the AIMS from most of the earlier motor measures that required specific positioning of an infant and extensive handling. Infants often become stressed when placed in testing positions unfamiliar to them such as vertical or ventral suspension, or when testing isolated items such as reflexes, muscle tone, or range of motion that require extensive handling and may constrain an infant's spontaneous motor behaviors. Because of this concern, during an AIMS assessment an infant is observed with minimal handling and no arbitrary stimuli or facilitation. Instead, infants move freely during the assessment, motivated by their environmental surroundings and with minimal handling by the assessor. Parents are encouraged to stay close to their infant during the assessment, and the assessor can observe unobtrusively from a distance if the infant is shy or upset. The infant sets the pace of the assessment with the assessor responding to an infant's cues rather than imposing specific postures or movements. The assessment is interrupted if an infant is anxious and is resumed only when the infant is composed. An infant's own toys may be used as motivators for movement; no specific toys, prompts, or conditions are required to assess movement. The goal of an AIMS assessment is to observe an infant's gross motor skills with minimal handling by the assessor and to provide specific scoring criteria to ensure standardization of scoring.

CONSTRUCTION OF THE AIMS

Development of the AIMS began with a literature review of existing instruments and descriptive narratives of early motor development to determine the functional sequences and variations that occur in early motor development (Amiel-Tison & Grenier, 1986; Bly, 1980; Saint-Anne Dargassies, 1986; Tscharnuter, 1982). Eighty-four items were generated based on these published descriptive narratives of early motor performance. Four separate sets of items were written, corresponding to four positions: prone, supine, sitting, and standing. An artist was hired to capture each item in a visual form. Each item consists of an artist's drawing of an infant doing a specific motor skill accompanied by a detailed description of the weight-bearing, posture, and antigravity movements observed in that position.

Meetings were held with pediatric physical therapists in the province of Alberta, Canada, to review the 84 items for appropriateness, content, and clinical importance. In addition, a mail inquiry was conducted of 291 members of the Pediatric Division of the Canadian Physiotherapy Association. Members were randomly sent copies of the prone items, the standing items, or the supine and sitting items. Each therapist was asked to rate each item on three criteria: (1) the importance of the item to gross motor development, (2) the likelihood that the infant would demonstrate the item during a 30-minute assessment, and (3) how easy it would be to observe the item descriptors. Participants were also asked to sort the items within each of the four position subsets as to their typical order of emergence and to give an age range within which each item would be observed in typically developing infants. Analyses of their responses resulted in the elimination of 17 items and revision of other item descriptions.

Initial placement (scaling) of the remaining 67 items along the continuum of motor development was accomplished using the therapists' averaged estimate of the ages of emergence for each item. In addition, the data from the item sorting task were subjected to a multidimensional scaling procedure to assess whether dimensions other than developmental sequencing were necessary to account for the therapists' responses. Only one dimension, motor maturation, was identified.

The next phase involved seeking expert opinion of the item sets. Six international experts in infant motor development attended a 2-day work session as part of the content validation process. The work session was comprised of four stages. First, the experts were each given a copy of the item sets and were asked to review them independently for clarity, significance, order, and inclusiveness. Second, the six experts were divided into two groups of three members each and asked to review in detail specific item sets. Each group was to (1) determine the accurate sequence of the items within the set, (2) remove inappropriate items from the set, and (3) add items, if necessary, to the set. The third stage involved combining the four sets of items on a maturational continuum. The experts were then asked to review the entire set of items for redundancies, sequencing of occurrence, and omissions. Finally, a group session was held to discuss administration and scoring issues in general.

The scale was further revised by the authors after this consultation process, and administrative guidelines were developed. Thirteen items were deleted, and five new items were constructed, resulting in a total of 59 items. A score sheet was developed for use in a feasibility test. Three pediatric physical therapists were hired and trained in the administration of the infant motor measure in preparation of the feasibility test.

Ninety-seven low-risk infants, age-stratified through the first 18 months of life and deemed to be typically developing, were recruited for the feasibility study through the Edmonton Board of Health well-baby clinics. These infants were assessed on the infant motor maturation scale by one of the three pediatric physical therapists. Their input generated recommendations concerning feasibility of observing the items as described, wording of administrative guidelines, and the format of the recording form.

Certain scaling models were tested on the feasibility data, including multidimensional scaling, Guttman scaling, and item response models. Although these analyses involved a small number of infants per age category, the items appeared to be measuring a single dimension (motor maturity), and the ordering of items on the developmental continuum largely confirmed what had been anticipated.

Following the collection of the feasibility data, seven items were deleted, and six new items added, resulting in a total of 58 items (21 prone items, 9 supine items, 12 sitting items, and 16 standing items) to be included for the reliability and validity testing. Key descriptors that must be observed for the infant to pass each item were identified and included on the score sheets. In preparation for the reliability and validity testing, guidelines for administration and scoring were developed.

The results of the reliability and validity testing are reported in Chapter 10. The interrater reliability, test-retest reliability, concurrent validity, and discriminative validity of the AIMS have been assessed. These tests revealed that the AIMS is reliable and valid in discriminating the motor performance of typically developing infants from that of at-risk infants and those with identified motor delay. It also captures small changes in motor skills due to maturation.

Once the AIMS was determined to be both reliable and valid, age- and sex-related norms were developed on the basis of assessing the motor performance of a cross-sectional sample of 2200 infants representative of all Albertan infants born between March 1990 and June 1992. The establishment of these norms permits the use of the AIMS as a discriminative index by providing for the identification of those infants whose performance is either delayed or aberrant in relation to their peers or the normative group. This normative database ensures that the performance of an individual child who is assessed with the AIMS is properly interpreted. The procedures used to collect the normative data are presented in Chapter 11. A reevaluation of the normative data was completed in 2014 and is described in Chapter 11.

In summary, the AIMS is a carefully constructed, theoretically sound, performance-based, norm-referenced, observational tool to assess the gross motor maturation of infants from 40 weeks postconception to independent walking. The 58 items of the AIMS incorporate the components of motor development that are deemed important by therapists for the evaluation and treatment of at-risk infants. The psychometric properties of the AIMS suggest that it is a psychometrically sound instrument appropriate to evaluate small increments of change in the motor development of infants. The normative data provide for the identification of those infants whose motor performance is delayed for their age. The AIMS is used internationally for teaching, clinical, and research purposes as a standardized psychometrically strong measure of infant gross motor abilities.

Prone Lying

Weight Bearing	Weight on hands, forearms, and chest
Posture	Elbows behind shoulders and close to body Hips and knees flexed
Antigravity Movement	Lifts head asymmetrically to 45° Cannot maintain head in midline

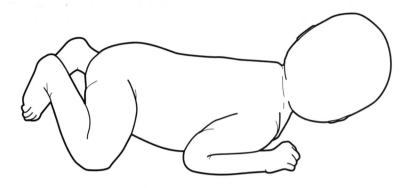

Rolling Supine to Prone Without Rotation

Weight Bearing	Weight on one side of body
Posture	Head up Trunk elongated on weight-bearing side Shoulder in line with pelvis
Antigravity Movement	Lateral head righting Rolling initiated from head, shoulder, or hip Trunk moves as one unit

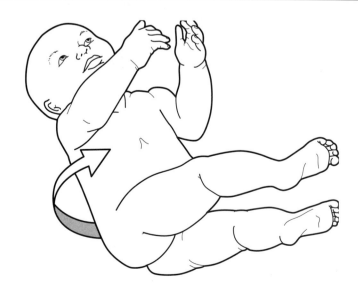

Sitting With Arm Support

Weight Bearing	Weight on buttocks, legs, and hands
Posture	Head up; shoulders elevated Hips flexed, externally rotated, and abducted Knees flexed Lumbar and thoracic spine rounded
Antigravity Movement	Maintains head in midline Supports weight on arms briefly

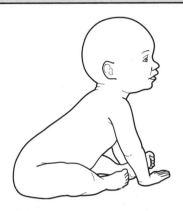

Cruising Without Rotation

Weight Bearing	Weight on feet Some arm support
Posture	Legs abducted and externally rotated Wide base of support Body faces forward
Antigravity Movement	Cruises sideways without rotation

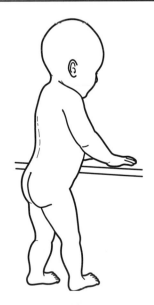

REFERENCES

American Academy of Pediatrics, Committee on Children with Disabilities. (2001). Developmental surveillance and screening for infants and young children. *Pediatrics, 108*(1), 192–195.

Amiel-Tison, C., & Grenier, A. (1986). *Neurological assessment during the first year of life*. Oxford University Press.

Bayley, N. (1969). *Bayley scales of infant development*. Psychological Corporation.

Bly, L. (1980). The components of normal movement during the first year of life. In D. Slaton (Ed.), *Development of movement in infancy* (pp. 85–123). Division of Physical Therapy, University of North Carolina.

Council on Children with Disabilities, Section on Developmental Behavioral Pediatrics, Bright Futures Steering Committee Medical Home Initiatives for Children with Special Needs Project Advisory Committee. (2006). Identifying infants and young children with developmental disorders in the medical home: An algorithm for developmental surveillance and screening. *Pediatrics, 118*(1), 405–420.

Effgen, S. K., & Howman, J. (2013). Child appraisal: Examination and evaluation. In S. K. Effgen (Ed.), *Meeting the physical therapy needs of children* (2nd ed., pp. 107–152). F. A. Davis.

Fanaroff, A. A., Hack, M., & Walsh, M. C. (2003). The NICHD Neonatal Research Network: Changes in practice and outcomes during the first 15 years. *Seminars in Perinatology, 27*(4), 281–287.

Folio, M. R., & Fewell, R. R. (1983). *Peabody developmental motor scales and activity cards: A manual*: DLM Teaching Resources.

Heineman, K. R., & Hadders-Algra, M. (2008). Evaluation of neuromotor function in infancy—a systematic review of available methods. *Journal of Developmental and Behavioral Pediatrics, 29*(4), 315–323.

Khan, L. (2019). Detecting early developmental delays in children. *Pediatric Annals, 48*(10), e381–e384.

Lee, S. K., Beltempo, M., McMillan, D. D., Seshia, M., Singhal, N., Dow, K., Azid, K., Piedboeuf, B., & Shah, P. S. (2020). Outcomes and care practices for preterm infants born at less than 33 weeks' gestation: A quality-improvement study. *Canadian Medical Association Journal, 192*(4), e81–e91.

Radecki, L., Sand-Loud, N., O'Connor, K. G., Sharp, S., & Olson, L. M. (2011). Trends in the use of standardized tools for developmental screening in early childhood: 2002-2009. *Pediatrics, 128*(1), 14–19.

Saint-Anne Dargassies, S. (1986). *The neuro-motor and psycho-affective development of the infant*. Elsevier.

Tscharnuter, I. (1982). Normal and abnormal sensorimotor development. In A. L. Scherzer, & I. Tscharnuter (Eds.), *Early diagnosis and therapy in cerebral palsy: A primer on infant developmental problems* (pp. 73–122). Marcel Dekker.

4

Administration Guidelines

AGE AND TYPE OF CLIENT

The purpose of the Alberta Infant Motor Scale (AIMS) is to assess the maturation of motor skills of infants from birth (40 weeks conception) to 18 months of age. The assessment process identifies the *components* of motor skills that can be observed during an infant's spontaneous movement choices. The appropriate use of the AIMS with infants in this age range depends on the reason for the assessment. If the purpose of the assessment is to *identify* infants who are exhibiting motor delays, the AIMS may be used with all infants ages term to 18 months, regardless of their movement strategies. An AIMS assessment may be used to determine if an infant's motor repertoire, at the time of assessment, represents typical motor skills, immature motor skills, delayed motor skills, or atypical motor patterns.

If the purpose of the assessment is to *evaluate* or monitor the maturation of an infant's motor skills over time, the AIMS may be used with infants 18 months or younger who are in one of the following categories:

1. Infants with typical motor development and no medical concerns.

   As with well-established growth parameters such as height and weight, the AIMS may be administered in well-baby clinics to provide information to health professionals and caregivers as to the progress of the infant's motor development over time. The normative data of the AIMS permit the comparison of an infant's motor development with an age-matched peer group by providing a percentile rank. The administration of the AIMS is useful in providing developmental information and feedback to caregivers about the motor performance of their infants over the first 18 months of life.

2. Infants with no predisposing factors in their medical histories but who have been identified as having suspect development in routine medical examinations.

   These infants are typically full-term infants who have experienced no complications in the pre-, peri-, or neonatal periods. Physicians or public health nurses often identify these infants in well-baby or immunization clinics. The AIMS may be used by these health professionals as an objective evaluation of the motor development of these infants, permitting the comparison of the infant's development to peers of the same age.

3. Infants considered to be at risk for developmental delay. Infants may be considered to be at risk because of adverse genetic, prenatal, perinatal, neonatal, postnatal, or environmental influences. Many infants in this category have received care in a neonatal intensive care unit and are subsequently followed in neonatal follow-up clinics. The majority of these infants are born preterm; full-term infants with medical problems during or after birth are also included in this category. The AIMS is useful to monitor the motor development of at-risk infants over time to identify those infants who are experiencing difficulty or delays in their motor development.

4. Infants with a specific diagnosis.

   The AIMS may also be used to monitor the maturation of motor skills of infants who have a specific diagnosis that includes *immature* motor development as one of its presenting signs. Examples of such diagnoses are fetal alcohol syndrome, Down syndrome, failure to thrive, bronchopulmonary dysplasia, and developmental delay. Infants with these diagnoses may exhibit immature or delayed acquisition of motor skills and often have muscle hypotonia. They demonstrate immature but typical patterns of movement, and the components of their motor skills may be captured by the descriptors of AIMS items.

The AIMS should not be used to evaluate the motor abilities of children older than 18 months whose motor skills are still at an infant level. The percentile rank tables cannot be used with these children to interpret a raw score. It is inappropriate to evaluate the motor abilities of older children on an infant scale of motor maturation even if their motor skills are at an infant level. Their motor performance needs to be evaluated using a measure that assesses their functional motor skills rather than components of infant motor skills.

The AIMS also should not be used to monitor the motor development over time of infants less than 18 months of age who use functional compensatory movement solutions because of limitations such as muscle spasticity, severe hypotonia, paralysis, and joint contractures. Although these infants often discover movement solutions that improve their function, this improvement will not be reflected in an AIMS score because they often use motor strategies that differ significantly from the components of movement described in the AIMS items. Infants with diagnoses such as spina bifida, arthrogryposis, spinal muscle atrophy, or cerebral palsy may improve their motor function by discovering unique movement patterns not included in descriptors of typical motor maturation. Their scores on the AIMS will remain unchanged even though their motor function improves. For example, infants with a diagnosis of spastic diplegia who have learned to pivot using only their arms cannot pass the pivot item on the AIMS unless their arms and legs move synchronously. Thus these infants cannot receive credit on the AIMS for their new functional motor skill. The AIMS is intended to evaluate the motor skills over time of infants with immature but typical patterns of movement and to compare their scores on the AIMS with scores collected on a representative sample of age-matched, normally developing infants.

OBSERVATIONAL APPROACH

The AIMS was designed as an observational assessment tool, requiring minimal handling of an infant by the examiner. Although facilitation and handling are often necessary elements of intervention strategies, they should be avoided during an AIMS assessment. Instead, an infant's spontaneous motor skills are observed without extensive handling by the examiner.

Pediatric therapists combine their observational and handling skills when they treat infants with movement challenges. They modify their intervention techniques in response to the reactions they observe in the infants; the techniques may include changing the environment, suggesting different play positions, and showing parents how to handle their infant. Although competent handling is part of effective treatment strategies for infants with motor disorders, handling may be detrimental during the assessment of an infant's motor skills. Traditional testing of developmental markers such as primitive reflexes, muscle tone, and righting and equilibrium reactions entails both extensive handling of an infant and the placement of the infant in arbitrary and stressful testing positions, such as vertical and horizontal suspension. This style of testing may upset an infant and result in a suboptimal response. In contrast, when a therapist observes an infant's spontaneous movement without extensive handling, the infant's integrated, functional movements may be observed in context. Itemized, fragmented testing may result in a narrow analysis of movement skills. The lack of one age-appropriate reaction or reflex may not be worrisome if an infant is moving in a typical manner. For example, an absent placing reaction in a 6-month-old infant is insignificant if age-appropriate motor skills are present. Concern arises when an infant's spontaneous movements are affected by the presence of a cluster of atypical components.

During an AIMS assessment the infant, not the examiner, initiates the motor skills described by the items. The examiner interacts with the infant to encourage the observation of specific AIMS items, but active facilitation of movement is avoided. Observation of an infant's spontaneous movements encourages the observation of both the positive and concerning aspects of an infant's motor repertoire. Traditional assessments of motor development often include the documentation of abnormal components of movement, such as the presence of an evoked asymmetric tonic neck reflex or ankle clonus. Testing components of movement in isolation may overemphasize negative findings, while observing an infant's spontaneous movements allows for the synthesis of both the positive and negative aspects of an infant's movement repertoire. If selective testing of reflexes, muscle tone, joint range of motion, etc., is necessary, it is recommended that they be performed after the completion of an AIMS assessment.

An observational assessment approach increases the social comfort level of an infant. Stranger anxiety is a typical stage of development for infants in the first year of life. Often an infant becomes upset when handled by a therapist, and this agitated state may prevent observation of an infant's optimal motor abilities. Although the observational approach is usually welcomed by parents and infants, therapists are sometimes initially uncomfortable with this assessment approach because they interpret it as a hands-off approach. During an AIMS assessment the therapist actively engages with an infant, encouraging movement in different postures and positions. Some handling may be required, especially with very young infants, but extensive handling and facilitation of movement should be avoided.

Evaluators

The AIMS may be performed by any health professional with a background in infant motor development and an understanding of the components of movement described for each AIMS item. An examiner needs to achieve an acceptable level of inter- and intrarater reliability in administering the AIMS to a variety of infants prior to using the AIMS for clinical or research purposes.

Time Requirements

Twenty to 30 minutes is usually the maximum time required to complete an AIMS assessment. A large portion of this time may be used for the infant to acclimate to the testing situation. Once an infant begins moving, a series of items is usually observed over a brief period.

Materials Needed

- Examining table for infants 0 to 4 months
- Mat or carpeted area for older infants; the mat should be firm enough that it does not impede the infant's ability to move
- Toys appropriate for infants 0 to 18 months
- A stable bench or chair to observe some of the pull to stand, standing, and cruising items in the standing subscale
- AIMS score sheet and graph

Setting

The assessment may be done in a clinic or in the home. With young infants, the assessment may be conducted on an examining table or other raised surface. After 4 months of age, infants are typically examined on a mat or carpeted area. The usual precautions should be taken to ensure the safety of the infant during an assessment.

Parent Involvement

The parent or caregiver is present during the assessment and undresses the infant. The infant should be awake, active, and content during the assessment. The examiner and parent interact with the infant to achieve and maintain this optimal state. If the infant is anxious or shy, the examiner may observe from a distance and guide the parent in positioning the infant to observe specific items.

Prompting

Certain items require positioning or physical prompting; these items are clearly specified in their descriptions. Minimal handling of the infant is encouraged. Visual and auditory prompts may be used by the examiner or parent as required. The examiner may interact and play with an infant to encourage a response, but physical facilitation of a movement is avoided.

If a specific prompt is required for an item, it is indicated in the item description. Younger infants who are not yet assuming the positions independently may be placed in the four different positions to assess their motor development. For example, an infant who does not yet assume the sitting position may be placed in this position to assess emerging sitting motor abilities; however, the examiner should not facilitate the motor abilities in any position.

Sequencing of the Assessment

It is not necessary to administer the entire scale. An infant is tested only on items most appropriate for the infant's developmental level in each subscale. Examiner discretion, parental reporting, and the infant's age determine the starting point on the scale for each infant.

Although an infant must be assessed in each of the four subscales, the assessment does not have to follow any particular sequence, and one subscale does not have to be completed before observing an infant's motor skills in another subscale. Instead, items from the four subscales are observed as an infant moves naturally in and out of positions. If an infant is too young to move independently in and out of the four subscale positions, the examiner or parent may place the infant in a position. Sometimes an infant is capable of moving from one position to another but is not motivated to do so during an assessment. For example, an infant 7 to 8 months old is often very active in prone and does not spend much time in supine. To observe the infant rolling from supine to prone, the parent or examiner may have to position the infant in supine.

Scoring

We encourage examiners to "put the scoresheet away" and score items at the end of an assessment, not during the assessment. In this way, an infant's movement repertoire is observed in context rather than tracking individual items on the scoresheet. It also allows both the examiner and the parents to be fully engaged with the infant, not the scoresheet. If, after completing the scoresheet, the examiner wants to confirm an infant's response for a certain item, that item can be observed again.

The score sheet consists of a line drawing for each item with key descriptors of postures or components of movements that *must* be observed for an infant to receive credit for the item. Chapters 5 through 8 provide detailed descriptions of the weight-bearing, posture, and antigravity movements associated with items in each of the four subscales (prone, supine, sit, and stand). The scoring system is a dichotomous choice for each item scored as either "observed" or "not observed"; no option exists for an infant to receive partial credit for an item that is emerging.

For each of the four subscales, the least mature and most mature item observed during the assessment are identified and scored "observed." The items between the least and most mature "observed" items in each position represent an infant's possible motor repertoire in that position, the "motor window" of an infant's current skills. Each item within this motor window is scored either "observed" or "not observed"; *all* items within the window must be scored. An item is scored "observed" only if the examiner observed the item as depicted in the line drawing and described by the key descriptors on the score sheet during the assessment. No item may be credited on the basis of developmental assumptions or parental reporting. Occasionally, items within an infant's motor window may have already been mastered and discarded. However, if any items are within the window and are not observed during the assessment, for whatever reason, they must be scored "not observed." Figs. 4.1 and 4.2 illustrate possible scoring sequences.

Sample Score Sheet 1
O = "Observed"
NO = "Not Observed"

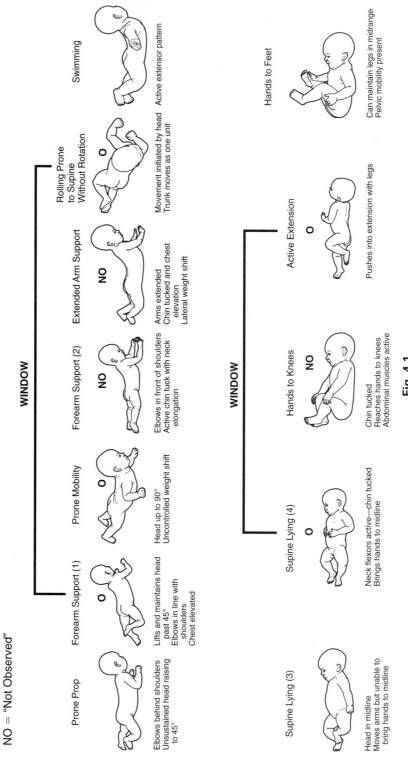

Fig. 4.1

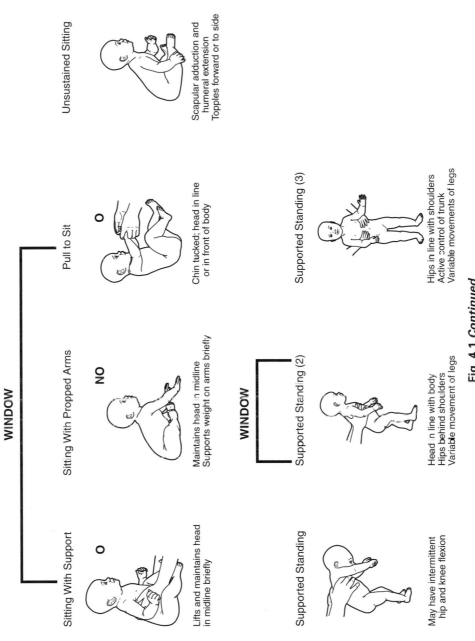

Sitting With Support

Lifts and maintains head in midline briefly

WINDOW

Sitting With Propped Arms

Maintains head in midline
Supports weight on arms briefly

Pull to Sit

Chin tucked; head in line or in front of body

Unsustained Sitting

Scapular adduction and humeral extension
Topples forward or to side

Supported Standing

May have intermittent hip and knee flexion

WINDOW

Supported Standing (2)

Head in line with body
Hips behind shoulders
Variable movement of legs

Supported Standing (3)

Hips in line with shoulders
Active control of trunk
Variable movements of legs

Fig. 4.1 *Continued*

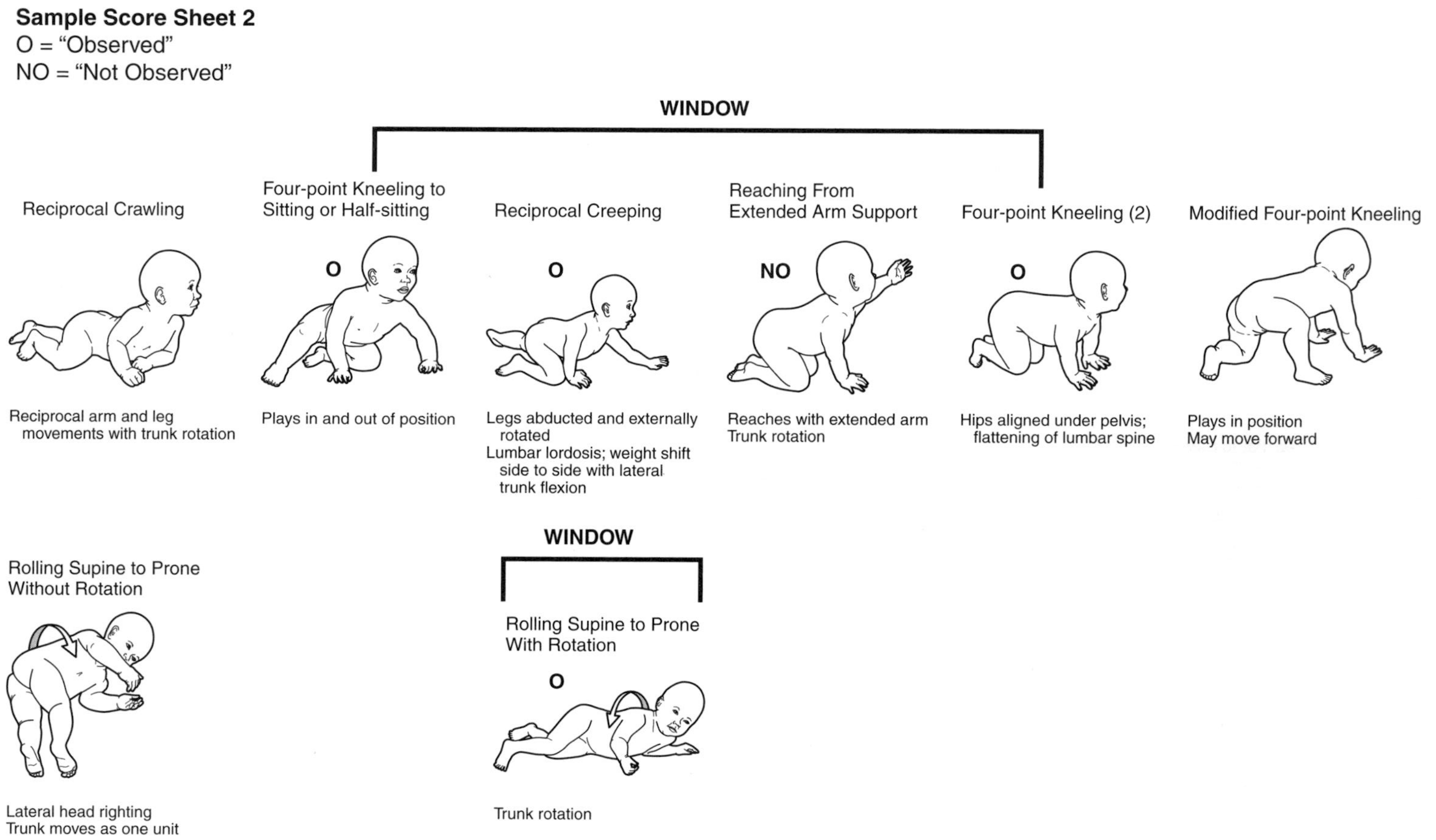

Sample Score Sheet 2
O = "Observed"
NO = "Not Observed"

WINDOW

Reciprocal Crawling

Reciprocal arm and leg
movements with trunk rotation

Four-point Kneeling to
Sitting or Half-sitting

O

Plays in and out of position

Reciprocal Creeping

O

Legs abducted and externally
rotated
Lumbar lordosis; weight shift
side to side with lateral
trunk flexion

Reaching From
Extended Arm Support

NO

Reaches with extended arm
Trunk rotation

Four-point Kneeling (2)

O

Hips aligned under pelvis;
flattening of lumbar spine

Modified Four-point Kneeling

Plays in position
May move forward

WINDOW

Rolling Supine to Prone
With Rotation

O

Trunk rotation

Rolling Supine to Prone
Without Rotation

Lateral head righting
Trunk moves as one unit

Fig. 4.2

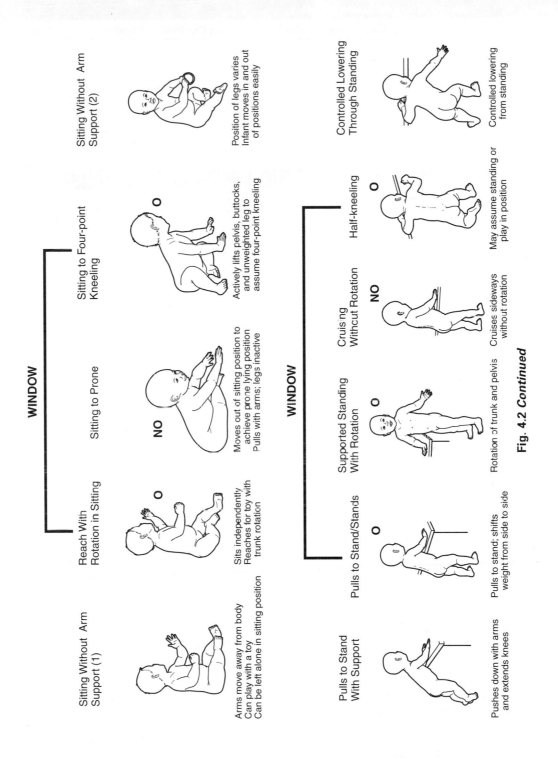

Sitting Without Arm Support (1)

Arms move away from body
Can play with a toy
Can be left alone in sitting position

WINDOW

Reach With Rotation in Sitting

O

Sits independently
Reaches for toy with trunk rotation

Sitting to Prone

NO

Moves out of sitting position to achieve prone lying position
Pulls with arms; legs inactive

Sitting to Four-point Kneeling

O

Actively lifts pelvis, buttocks, and unweighted leg to assume four-point kneeling

Sitting Without Arm Support (2)

Position of legs varies
Infant moves in and out of positions easily

Pulls to Stand With Support

Pushes down with arms and extends knees

WINDOW

Pulls to Stand/Stands

O

Pulls to stand; shifts weight from side to side

Supported Standing With Rotation

O

Rotation of trunk and pelvis

Cruising Without Rotation

NO

Cruises sideways without rotation

Half-kneeling

O

May assume standing or play in position

Controlled Lowering Through Standing

Controlled lowering from standing

Fig. 4.2 *Continued*

TABLE 4.1   Scoring: Sample Score Sheet 1

	Previous Items Credited	Items Credited in Window	Subscale Score
Prone	3	3	6
Supine	3	2	5
Sit	0	2	2
Stand	1	1	2
	Total Score 15		

TABLE 4.2   Scoring: Sample Score Sheet 2

	Previous Items Credited	Items Credited in Window	Subscale Score
Prone	15	3	18
Supine	8	1	9
Sit	8	2	10
Stand	4	3	7
	Total Score 44		

No minimum or maximum number of trials is necessary for scoring. The number of trials is dependent on the ability level of the infant and the allotted assessment time. For example, an infant who is just beginning to move spontaneously from a sitting to a prone position may initiate the movement many times before successfully completing it. If the examiner believes the infant is capable of completing the motor skill, the infant may be encouraged to attempt the movement a number of times. Sometimes it is necessary to leave an item and return to it later during the assessment. An assessment should not take longer than 30 minutes; if during this time an infant is happy and active and still has failed to perform a specific item, it is concluded that the item is not in the infant's motor repertoire.

Sometimes bidirectional motor items such as rolling, pivoting, and cruising are observed in only one direction, especially if it is a new skill for the infant. If the movement pattern meets the item descriptors, and if the examiner has no concerns about symmetry during the assessment process, the item may be credited even though it is observed in only one direction. However, if the examiner has overall concerns about asymmetry during the assessment, the item should be scored "not observed."

To determine an infant's total AIMS score, the four subscale scores (prone, supine, sitting, and standing) are calculated. Each item below the least mature item observed in each subscale is credited 1 point. Each "observed" item in the infant's motor window is credited 1 point. The sum of the credited points is the subscale score for each of the four

positions. The sum of the four subscale scores yields the infant's total score. See Tables 4.1 and 4.2 for scoring of the two example scoresheets (see Figs. 4.1 and 4.2).

In summary, to calculate a score:

1. Identify the least mature "observed" item in each subscale.
2. Identify the most mature "observed" item in each subscale.
3. The items between these two items are considered to be the infant's "motor window."
4. Score each item in the "window" as either "observed" or "not observed."
5. Credit 1 point to each item below the least mature "observed" item.
6. Credit 1 point to each item scored "observed" within the infant's "window."
7. Sum the points to obtain a subscale score.
8. Sum the four subscale scores to compute a total AIMS score.

PLOTTING THE SCORES

A graph is provided to plot the infant's total AIMS score (see Appendix I). From this graph, the examiner may determine the percentile ranking of the infant's motor performance compared with the normative age-matched sample of infants. To obtain an infant's percentile ranking, the infant's age, in months and weeks, is calculated using the following method:

Example 1

	Year	Month	Day
Date of Assessment	2020	12	10
Date of Birth	2020	4	5
Age at Assessment		8	5

Example 2

	Year	Month	Day
		13	40
Date of Assessment	~~2020~~	~~2~~	~~10~~
Date of Birth	2019	9	30
Age at Assessment		4	10

In Example 2, the value of the denominator for the month and day columns is larger than the numerator values because the values span two different years. For calculation purposes 12 months are moved from the year column (2020) making the month column equal to 14 months. Then one month is moved from the month column to the day assessment column resulting in 13 months 40 days. By convention each month contains 30 days, and each year contains 12 months. For an infant born at less than 37 weeks of gestation, corrected age is calculated by subtracting the days of prematurity from the age at assessment. Days of prematurity are calculated by subtracting the child's gestational age (in weeks) from 40 weeks (full term).

The infant's age is located on the horizontal axis of the graph, and the infant's total AIMS score is located on the vertical axis. A perpendicular line is drawn from each of these points; the percentile ranking of the infant's score may be determined from the point of intersection of these two lines. The information derived from plotting the child's score on the graph yields a single-point estimation of the child's percentile ranking. For example, if an infant who is 4 months, 1 week old receives a total AIMS score of 13, the percentile ranking on the graph would occur just below the 25th percentile.

The percentile ranking may also be determined by consulting Appendix II. The column that contains the infant's age is located. The infant's score is located in the raw score column. The percentile rank located at the intersection of the infant's raw score and the age group represents the percentile rank compared with the scores of infants in the same age grouping. Because the percentile ranks listed in Appendix II have been averaged over the entire age month,

it is important to recognize that the listed percentiles are less accurate for infants whose ages fall at the extremes of the age grouping, such as an infant who is 4 months, 1 day old or an infant who is 4 months, 28 days old.

The percentile ranking indicates what proportion of the normative sample of infants of the same age obtained a similar score. For example, a 60th percentile ranking for a 4-month-old infant indicates that 60% of the infant's peers obtained a score equal to or less than that obtained by the assessed infant and that only 40% of similar infants obtained a higher score. The higher the percentile ranking, the less likely that the infant is demonstrating a delay in motor development. For instance, an 80th or 90th percentile ranking clearly indicates that the infant's total score is equal to or greater than 80% or 90% of peers, with only 10% or 20% of peers obtaining a higher score. The interpretation of a lower percentile is less clear. Longitudinal monthly follow-up of healthy full-term infants' AIMS scores revealed that the infants did not maintain the same percentile rank over time and that some infants had one or more scores below the recommended cutoffs (Darrah et al., 1998). The AIMS is not a diagnostic test, and decisions regarding an infant's status and type of follow-up should be made in conjunction with other assessment information and parents' concerns. The predictive validity of AIMS scores is discussed in Chapter 9.

CONCLUSION

The AIMS is an observational assessment, where an infant's motor repertoire is observed in prone, supine, sitting, and standing positions. The assessment can be used from 0 to 18 months, with age-appropriate skills assessed of the infant observed through play. Therapists need to allow time for an infant to feel comfortable in the environment and, where appropriate, involve parents to ensure the infant is in an ideal state (i.e., awake, not crying, and playful). The AIMS can be used in a wide variety of patient populations, but the purpose of the assessment may vary.

REFERENCE

Darrah, J., Redfern, L., Maguire, T. O., Beaulne, A. P., & Watt, J. (1998). Intra-individual stability of rate of gross motor development in full-term infants. *Early Human Development, 52*(2).

5

Prone Subscale

The prone subscale contains 21 items. Each item consists of an artist's drawing of an infant accompanied by a photograph of a baby performing the movement. A detailed description of the weight-bearing, posture, and antigravity movements observed in each position is included with each item. These descriptions are more detailed than the key descriptors provided on the score sheet. The examiner should refer to the more detailed descriptions of the item for clarification of the weight-bearing, posture, and antigravity movements associated with each item. To receive credit for an item, the infant must exhibit all of the key descriptors noted on the score sheet.

The examiner may place a very young infant in the prone position. However, for older infants who are moving across the four subscales spontaneously, no physical handling is required to score the prone items. If an infant is walking independently and not creeping very often,

try to observe *Reciprocal Creeping (2),* the last item in the prone subscale, through play. The item can then be scored "observed", and the infant will receive credit for all items in prone.

Each item is accompanied by a graph depicting the percentage of infants in the normative sample for each age category that received credit for the particular item. On each graph, the *x*-axis indicates the age in months, and the *y*-axis represents the percentage of infants receiving credit for the item. A solid line has been drawn to indicate the age at which 50% of infants received credit for the item. A dotted line has been drawn at the age at which 90% of infants successfully completed the item. For example, in the *prone mobility* item, 50% of 3-month-old infants and 90% of 4-month-old infants successfully performed this item. These graphs provide information on the frequency distribution of the age of attainment of each skill.

Prone Lying (1)

Weight Bearing	Weight on cheek, hands, forearms, and upper chest
Posture	Head rotated to one side Physiological flexion Arms close to body; elbows flexed
Antigravity Movement	Turns head to clear nose from surface

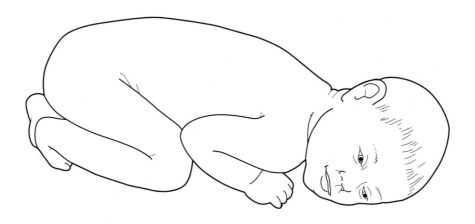

Prone lying (1)

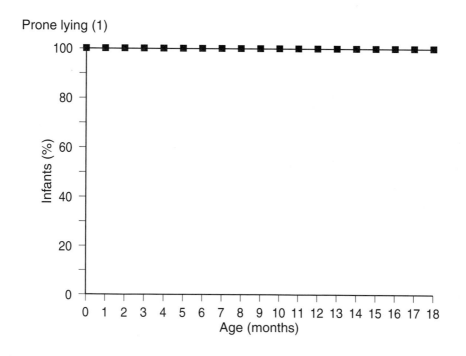

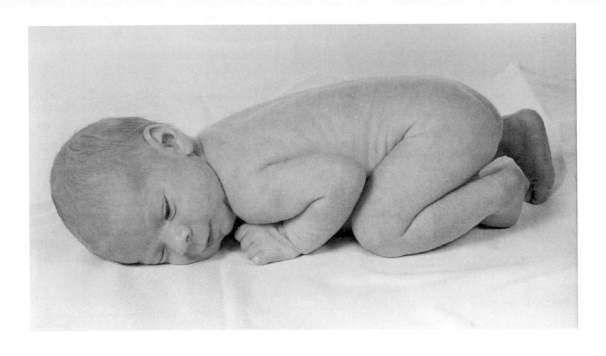

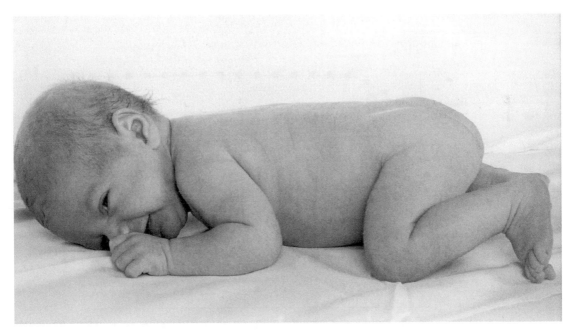

Prone Lying (2)

Weight Bearing	Weight on hands, forearms, and chest
Posture	Elbows behind shoulders and close to body Hips and knees flexed
Antigravity Movement	Lifts head asymmetrically to 45° Cannot maintain head in midline

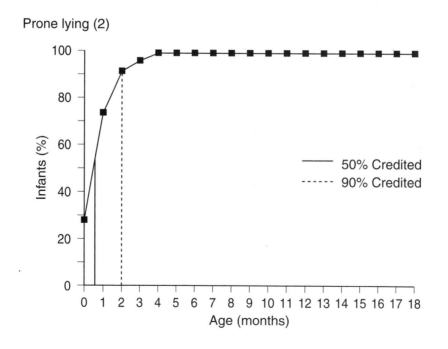

Prone lying (2)

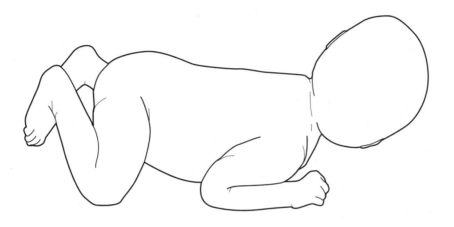

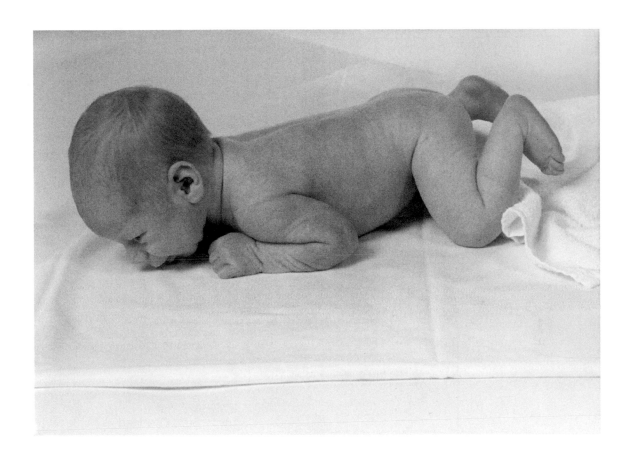

Prone Prop	
Weight Bearing	Weight on hands, forearms, and chest
Posture	Shoulders slightly abducted Elbows behind shoulders Hip and knees flexed
Antigravity Movement	Raises head to 45° Turns head
The infant is able to lift the head to 45° in the midline; this position may not be maintained indefinitely.	

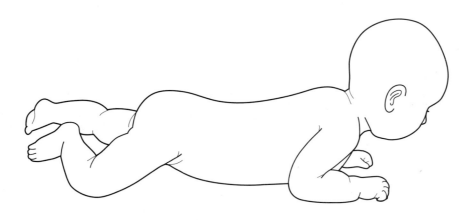

Prone prop

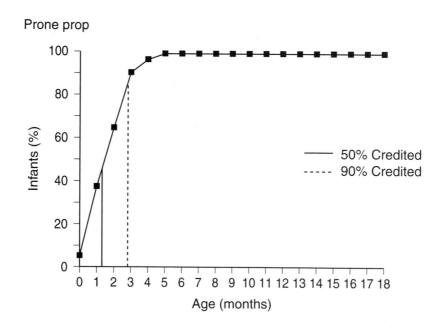

—— 50% Credited
- - - - 90% Credited

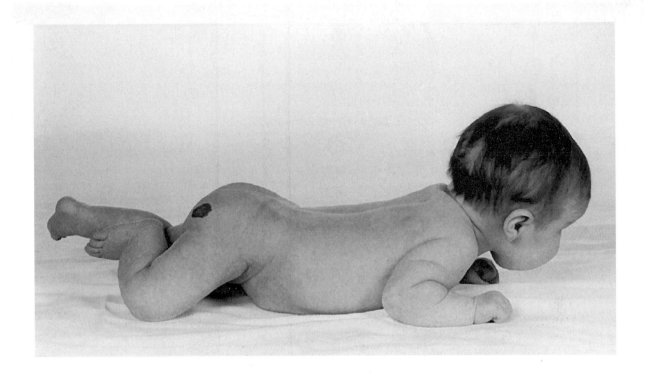

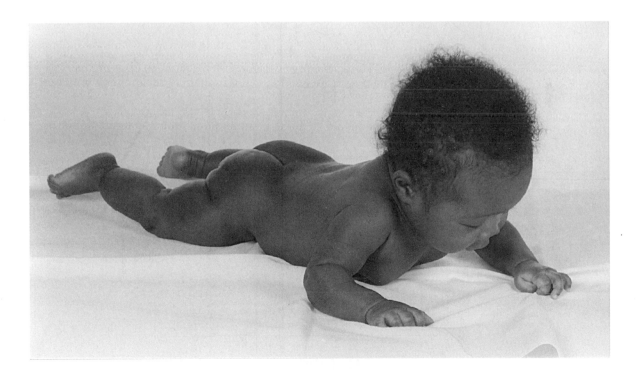

Forearm Support (1)

Weight Bearing	Weight symmetrically distributed on forearms and trunk
Posture	Shoulders abducted Elbows in line with shoulders Hips abducted and externally rotated Knees flexed
Antigravity Movement	Pushes against surface to raise head Lifts and maintains head past 45° Chest elevated

To pass this item the elbows must not be behind the shoulders; they may be beyond the shoulders. The infant may play with the feet together in this position. The head does not have to be maintained at 90°. Active chin tuck is not present.

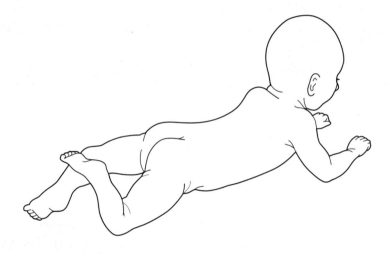

Forearm support (1)

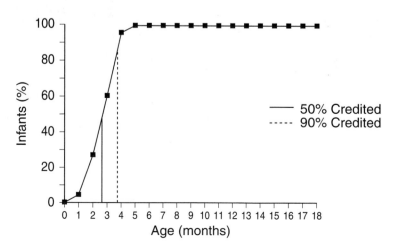

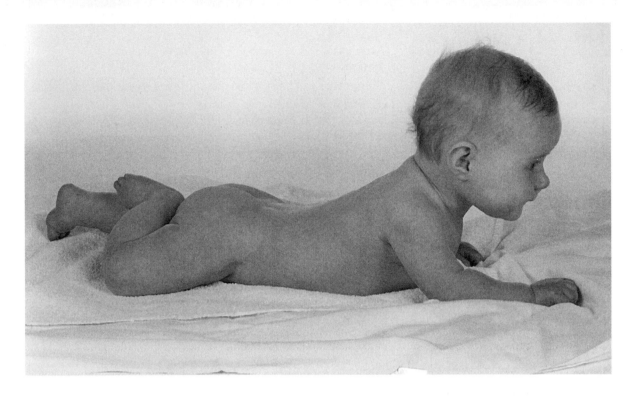

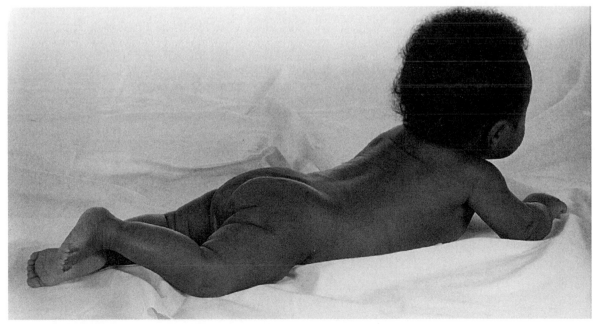

Prone Mobility

Weight Bearing	Weight on forearms, abdomen, and thighs
Posture	Head to 90° Forearm support or immature extended arm support Hips abducted
Antigravity Movement	Uncontrolled weight shift onto one arm; there may or may not be any displacement of the trunk
This item represents the infant's early attempts at weight shift in prone position.	
Prompt: May place toys appropriately to observe antigravity movements.	

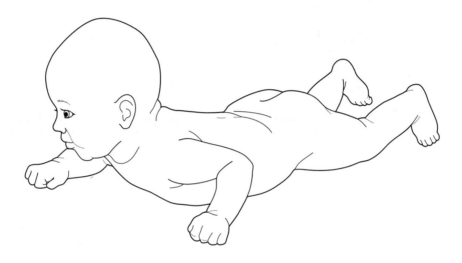

Prone mobility

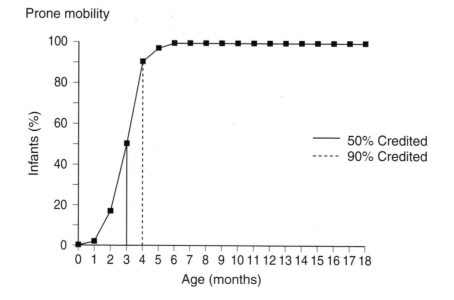

50% Credited
90% Credited

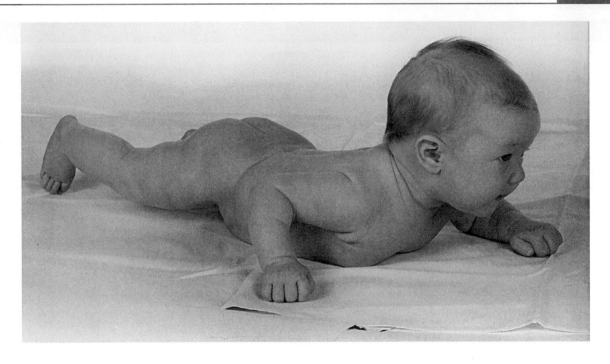

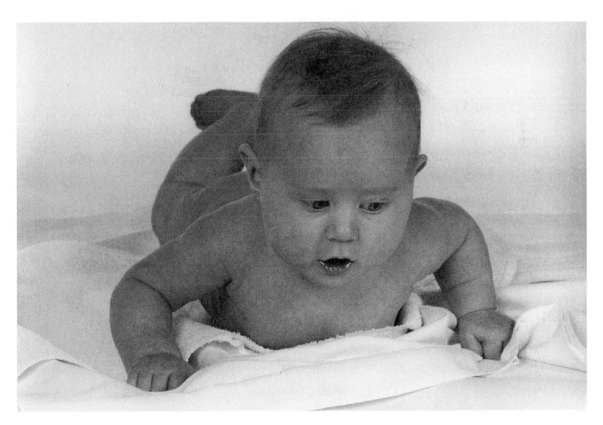

Forearm Support (2)

Weight Bearing	Weight on forearms, hands, and abdomen
Posture	Elbows in front of shoulders Hips abducted and externally rotated
Antigravity Movement	Raises and maintains head in midline Active chin tuck and neck elongation Chest elevated

The elbows must be in front of the shoulders to pass this item. The shoulders may be either abducted or in a more neutral position. The infant will often actively flex and extend the knees in this position. This item represents more mature head control than does the previous forearm support.

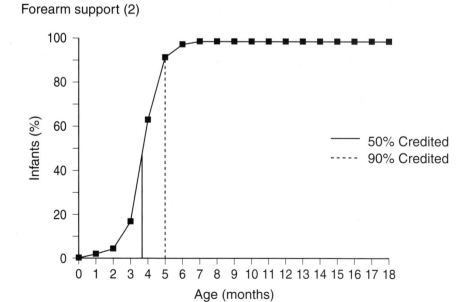

Forearm support (2)

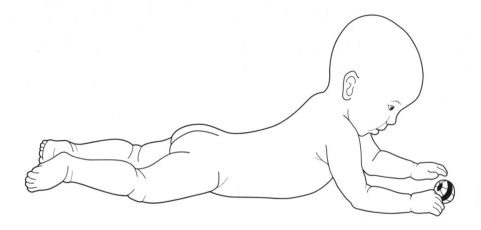

50% Credited
90% Credited

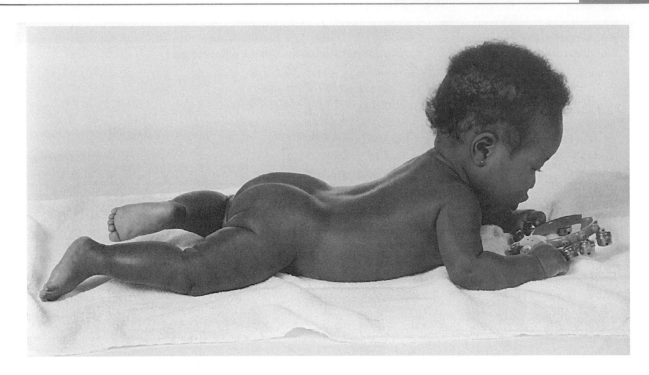

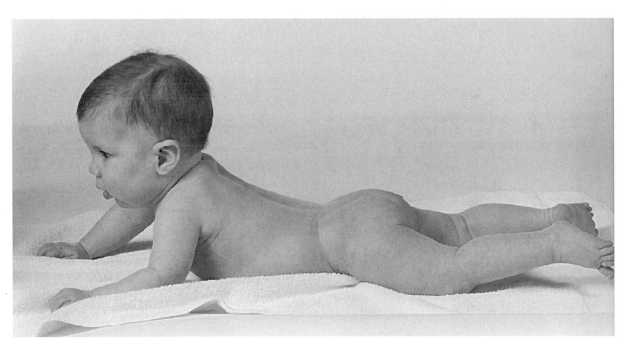

Extended Arm Support

Weight Bearing	Weight on hands, lower abdomen, and thighs
Posture	Arms extended Elbows in front of shoulders Legs approaching neutral position
Antigravity Movement	Chin tucked and chest elevated Flexion and extension of knees; may play with feet together Lateral weight shift
The infant may also push backward in this position.	

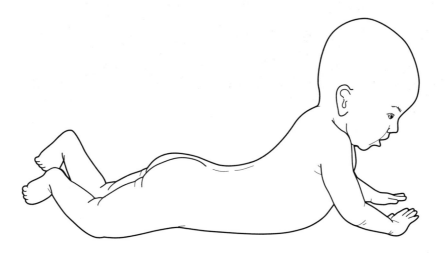

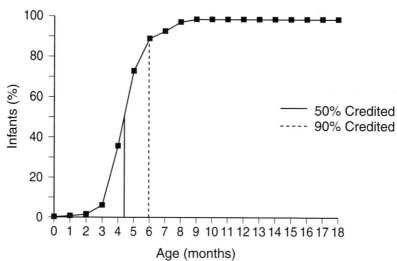

Extended arm support

50% Credited
90% Credited

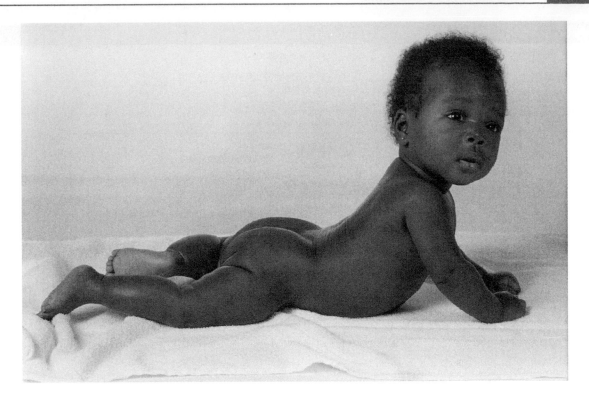

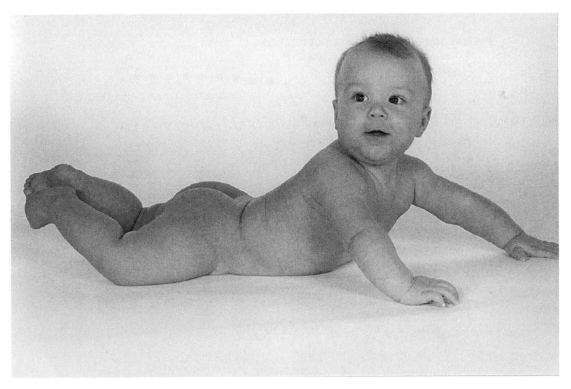

Rolling Prone to Supine Without Rotation

Weight Bearing	Weight on one side of body
Posture	Shoulder in line with pelvis Trunk extension
Antigravity Movement	Movement initiated by head Rolls prone to supine without trunk rotation

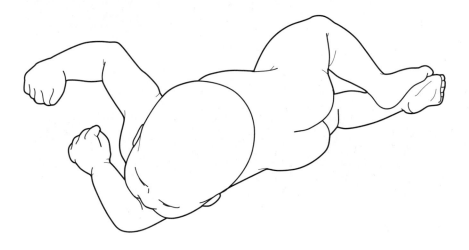

Rolling prone to supine without rotation

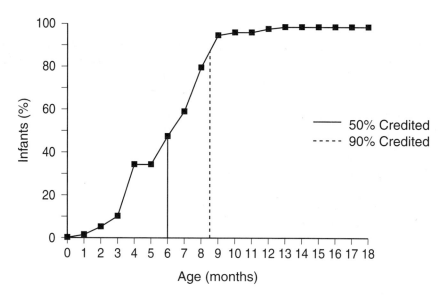

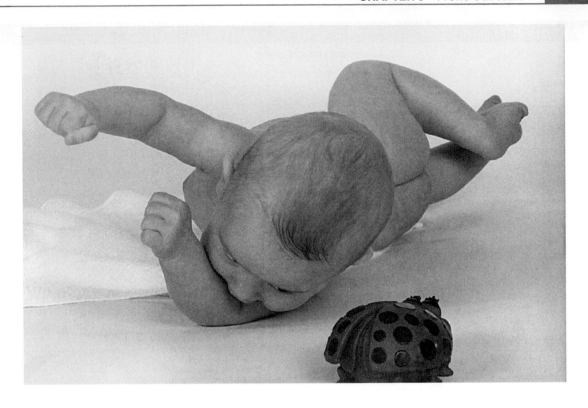

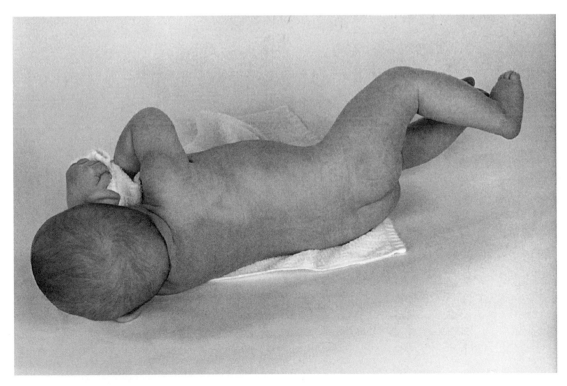

Swimming

Weight Bearing	Weight on abdomen
Posture	Symmetrical Scapulae adducted Arms abducted, externally rotated Legs abducted and extended Lumbar spine extended
Antigravity Movement	Raises head and arms or legs, or both, from surface Active extensor pattern

The infant may rock forward, backward, or side to side. There is no forward motion of the body, and sometimes the extensor activity is seen only in the arms or the legs. There should always be some active extension observed in the trunk.

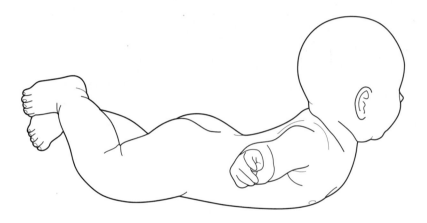

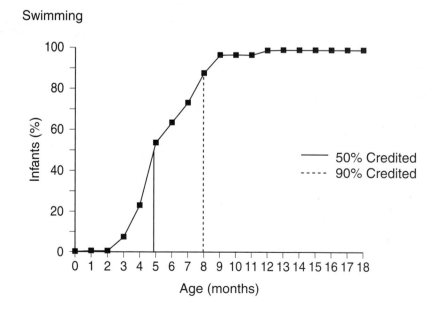

Swimming

50% Credited
90% Credited

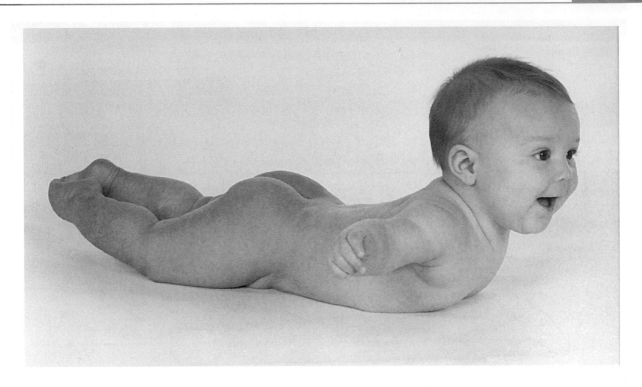

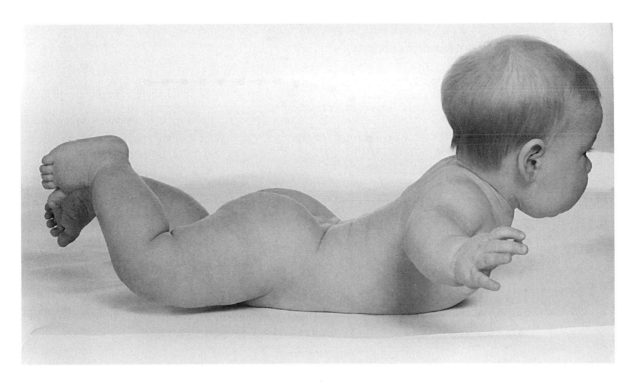

Reaching From Forearm Support

Weight Bearing	Weight on one forearm, hand, and abdomen
Posture	Forearm support Legs approaching neutral position
Antigravity Movement	Active weight shift to one side Controlled reach with free arm
This item represents a controlled reach; the infant does not lose balance as the arm reaches.	
Prompt: Object placed in midline or laterally to observe antigravity movements.	

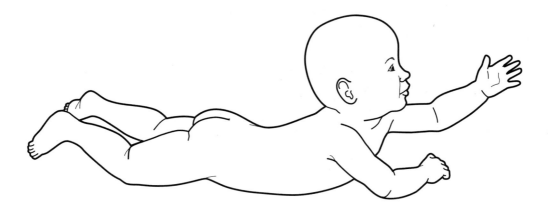

Reaching from forearm support

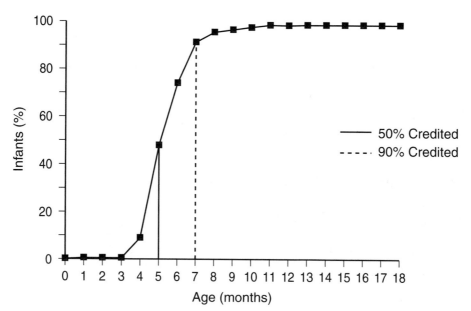

50% Credited
90% Credited

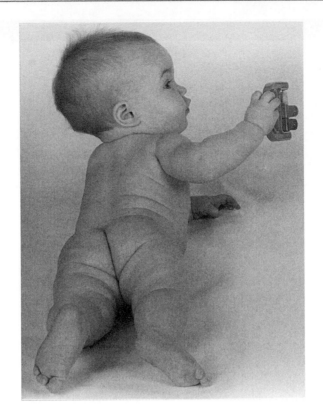

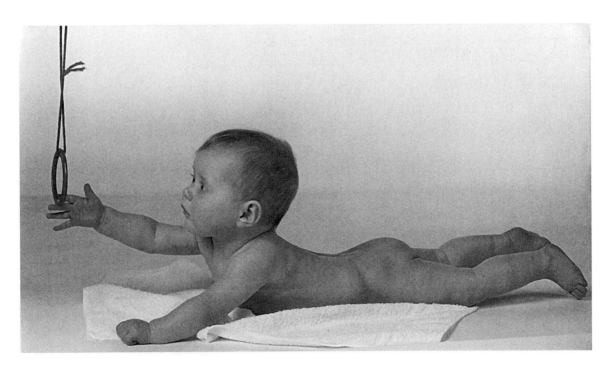

Pivoting

Weight Bearing	Weight on trunk, arms, and hands
Posture	Head to 90° Legs abducted and externally rotated
Antigravity Movement	Pivots Movement in arms and legs Lateral trunk flexion

To pass this item, the infant must use both arms and legs to pivot.

Prompt: Place toy laterally to initiate movement.

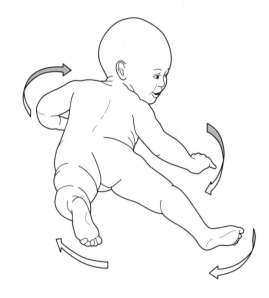

Pivoting

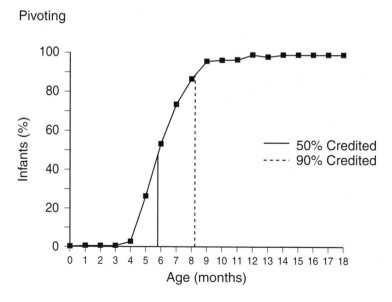

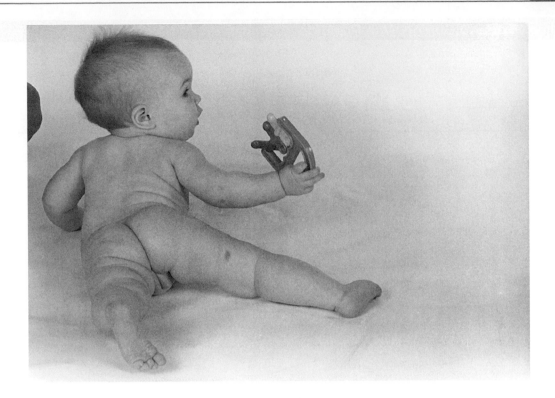

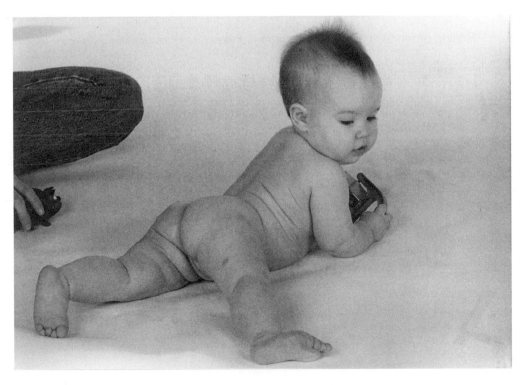

Rolling Prone to Supine With Rotation	
Weight Bearing	Weight on one side of body
Posture	Shoulder not in line with pelvis Trunk rotation
Antigravity Movement	Movement initiated by shoulder, pelvis, or head Trunk rotation

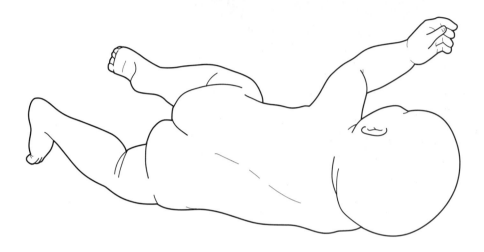

Rolling prone to supine with rotation

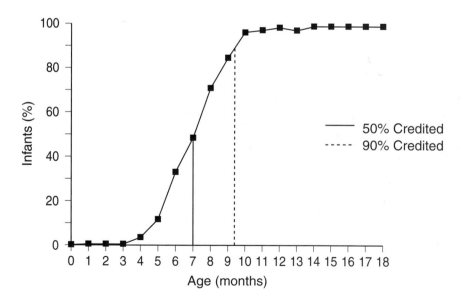

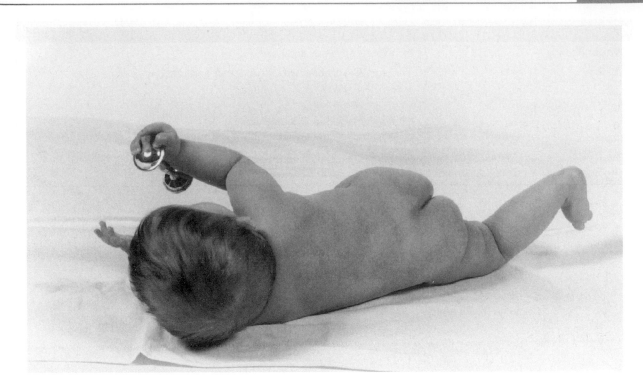

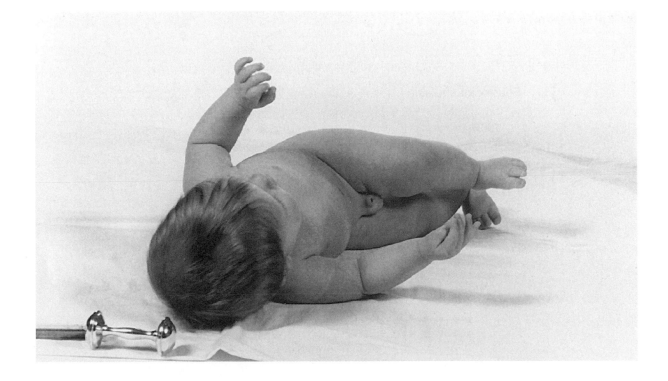

Four-Point Kneeling (1)

Weight Bearing	Weight on hands and knees
Posture	Legs flexed, abducted, and externally rotated Lumbar lordosis
Antigravity Movement	Maintains position May rock back and forth or diagonally May propel self forward by falling

This item is characterized by the immature posture of hip abduction. The shoulders may be internally rotated or in a neutral position. The infant need not be observed rocking to pass this item.

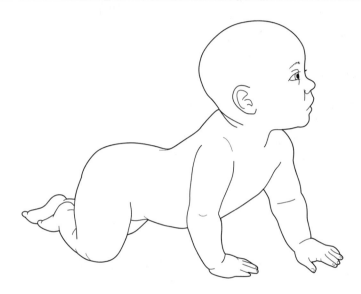

Four-point kneeling (1)

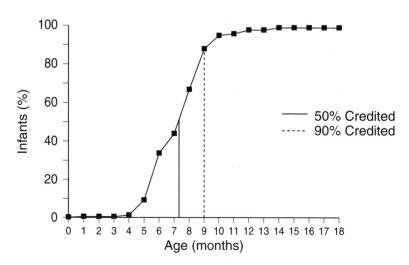

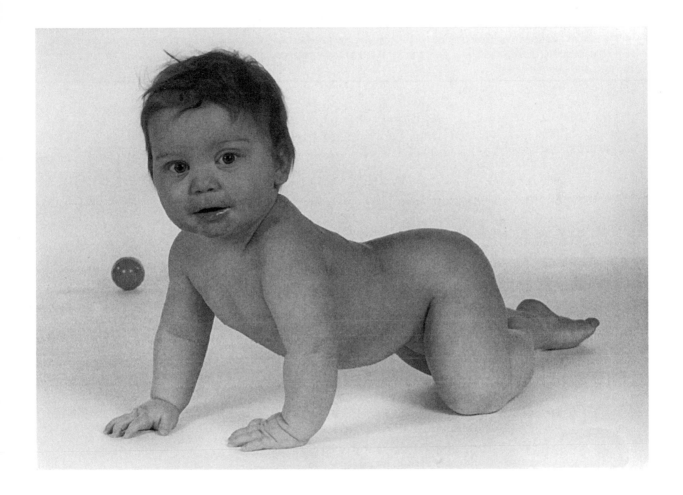

Propped Lying on Side

Weight Bearing	Weight on elbow, forearm, leg, and one side of trunk
Posture	Lateral head righting Lateral trunk flexion Upper leg flexed and adducted or abducted
Antigravity Movement	Dissociation of legs Shoulder stability Uses upper arm for reaching Rotation within body axis

The posture of the upper leg may change from hip abduction to adduction; the important features are shoulder stability and at least partial dissociation of one leg from the other. The infant may stay in this position only momentarily and move in and out of it often.

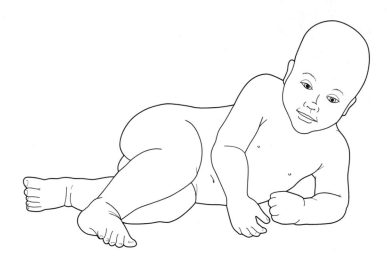

Propped on side

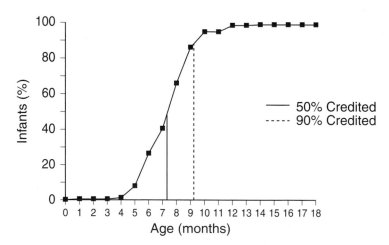

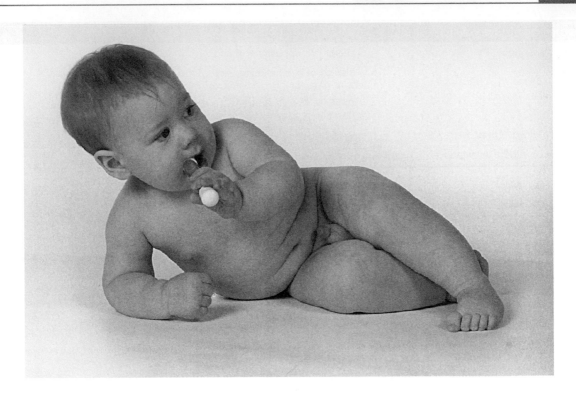

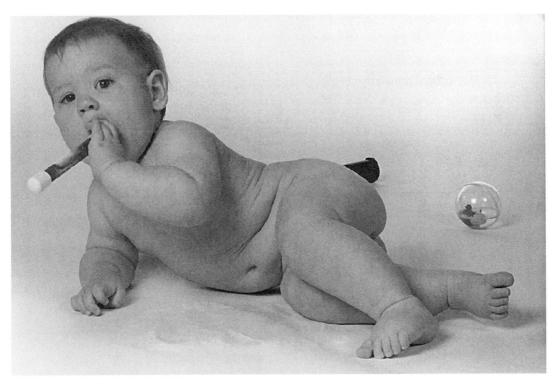

Reciprocal Crawling	
Weight Bearing	Weight on opposite arm and leg
Posture	Flexion of one hip, extension of the other Arm flexion Head to 90° Rotation in trunk
Antigravity Movement	Reciprocal arm and leg movements with trunk rotation
Movement in both arms and legs must be observed.	

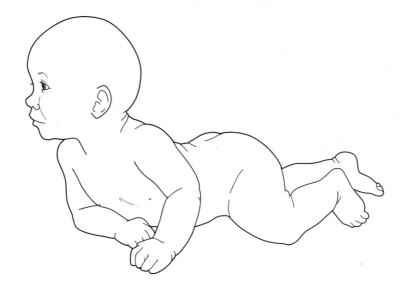

Reciprocal crawling

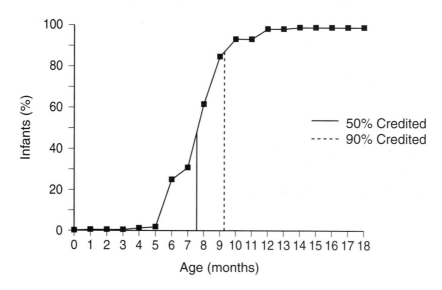

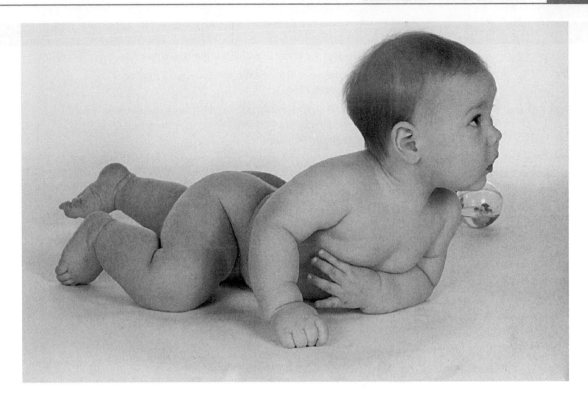

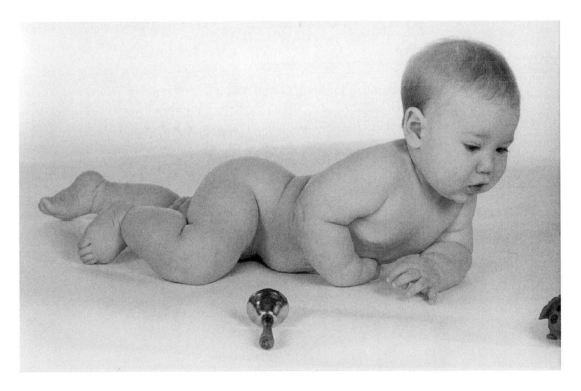

Four-Point Kneeling to Sitting or Half-Sitting

Weight Bearing	Weight on hands, leg, and foot on one side of body and other foot
Posture	Weight-bearing leg flexed and externally rotated Arms abducted
Antigravity Movement	Weight shift with elongation of trunk on weight-bearing side Plays in and out of position May get to sitting

The infant does not have to achieve sitting to pass this item; the midposition may follow four-point kneeling. Controlled movement of the pelvis is present.

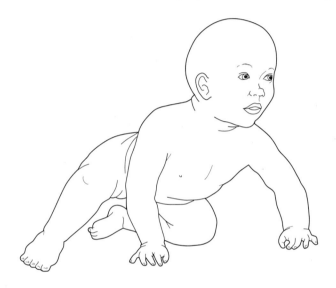

Four-point kneeling to sitting or half-sitting

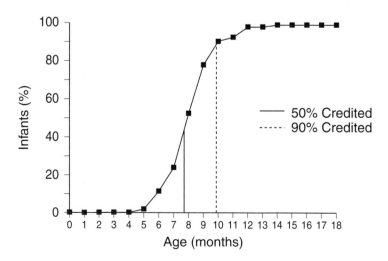

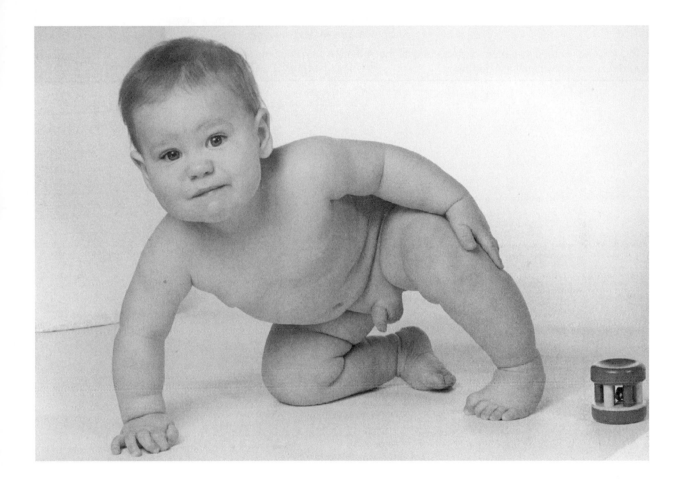

Reciprocal Creeping (1)

Weight Bearing	Weight on opposite hand and knee
Posture	Arms abducted Legs abducted and externally rotated Lumbar lordosis
Antigravity Movement	Weight shift side to side with lateral trunk flexion Reciprocal arm and leg movements

This is an early creeping pattern characterized by the immature posture of the legs and lack of trunk rotation. The infant must move forward to pass this item.

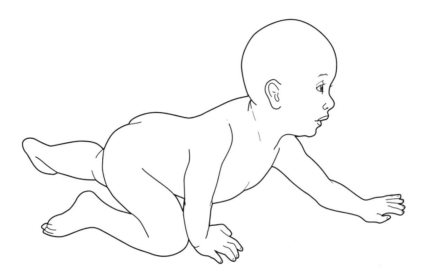

Reciprocal creeping (1)

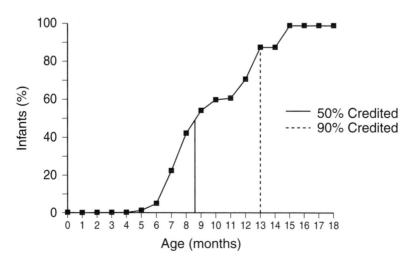

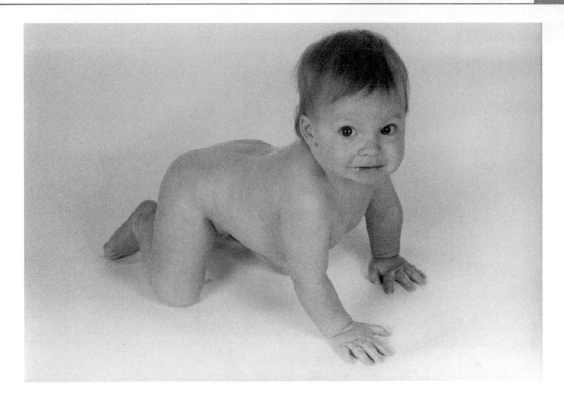

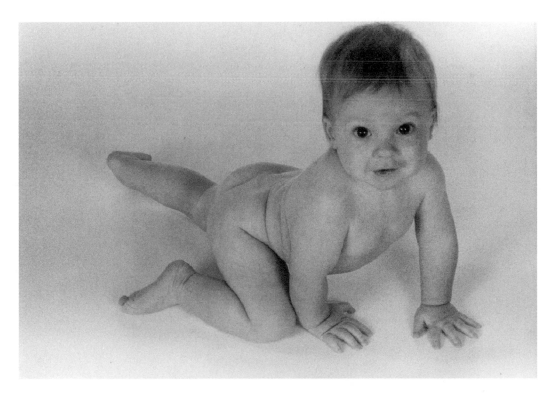

Reaching From Extended Arm Support

Weight Bearing	Weight on knees and one hand
Posture	Modified four-point kneeling with one arm off surface Weight-bearing arm extended
Antigravity Movement	Reaches with extended arm Rotation of head, shoulders, and trunk Weight-bearing arm may flex minimally

Prompt: May place toys appropriately to observe antigravity movements.

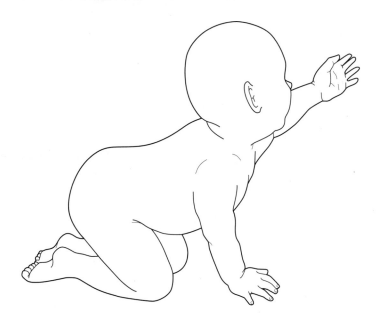

Reaching from extended arm support

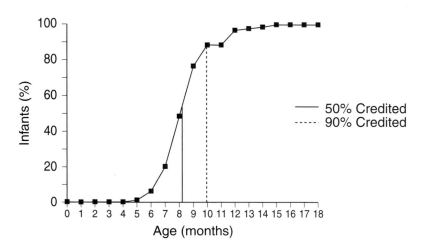

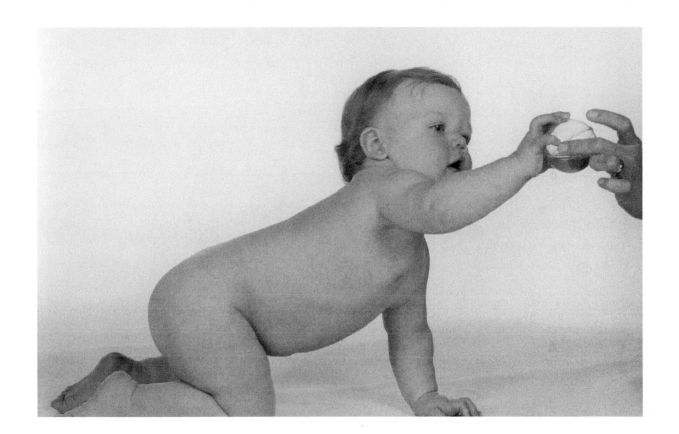

Four-Point Kneeling (2)

Weight Bearing	Weight on hands and knees
Posture	Legs flexed, hips aligned under pelvis Flattening of lumbar spine
Antigravity Movement	Abdominal muscles active Rocks back and forth and diagonally May propel self forward

This item is characterized by the mature posture of the hips aligned under the pelvis. The infant should either rock or creep forward to pass this item.

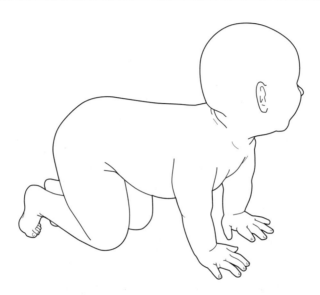

Four-point kneeling (2)

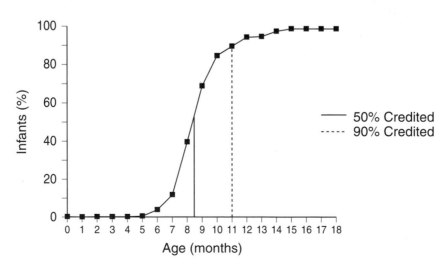

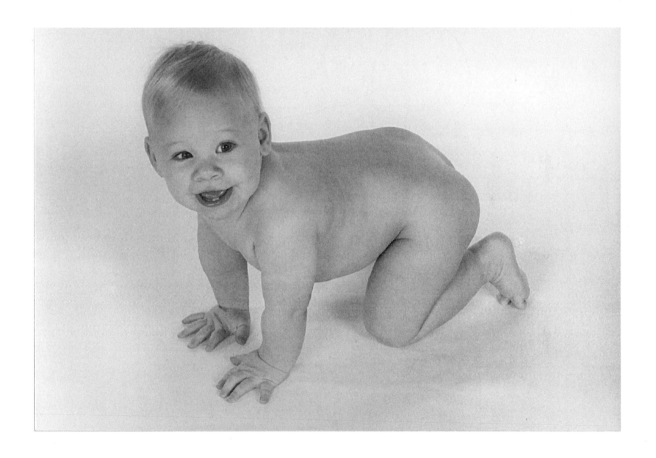

Modified Four-Point Kneeling

Weight Bearing	Weight on hands, one knee, and opposite foot
Posture	Modified quadruped position; one leg flexed at hip so that foot is planti-grade
Antigravity Movement	Plays in position May move forward

The flexed hip may be aligned under the pelvis or externally rotated. This is not a transitional movement to independent standing. It represents a variation of the four-point kneeling position.

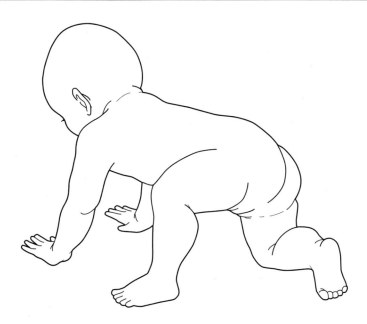

Modified four-point kneeling

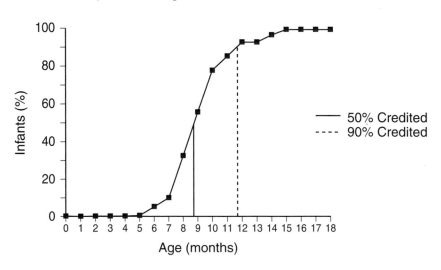

Age (months)

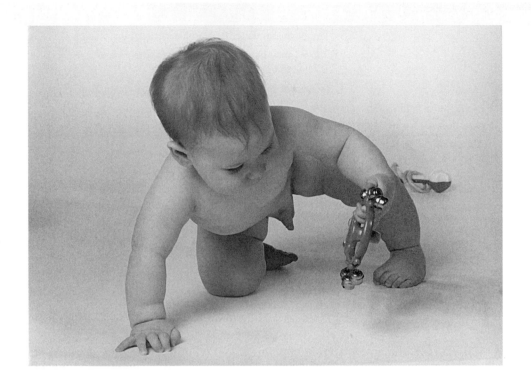

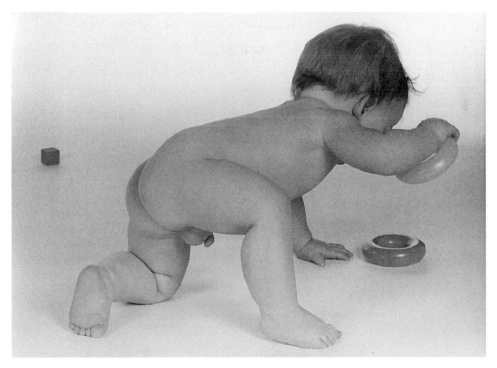

Reciprocal Creeping (2)

Weight Bearing	Weight on opposite hand and knee
Posture	Elbows and knees aligned under shoulders and hips Lumbar spine flat
Antigravity Movement	Reciprocal arm and leg movements with trunk rotation

This creeping pattern is characterized by the mature posture of the legs and trunk rotation. Lumbar lordosis is not present.

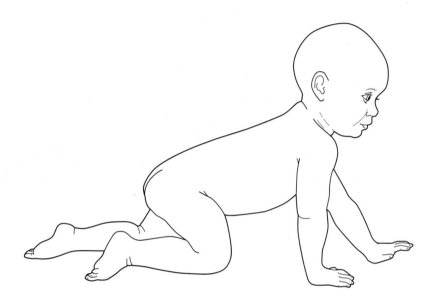

Reciprocal creeping (2)

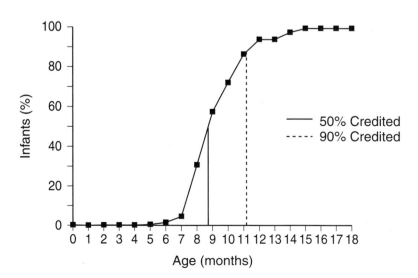

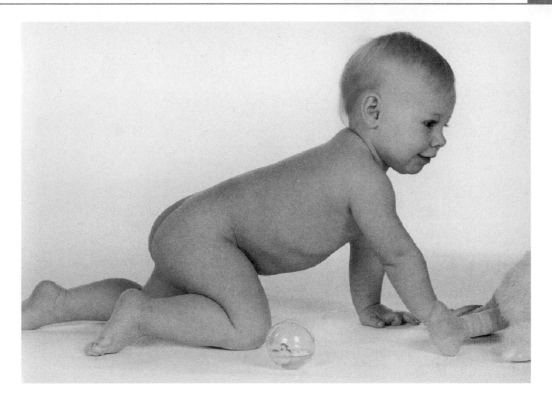

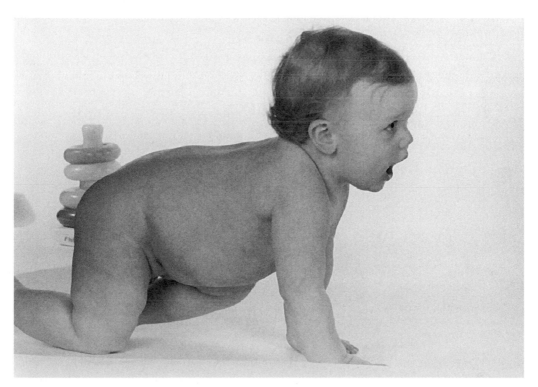

6

Supine Subscale

The supine subscale contains nine items. Each item consists of an artist's drawing of an infant accompanied by a photograph of a baby performing the movement. A detailed description of the weight-bearing, posture, and antigravity movements observed in each position is included with each item. These descriptions are more detailed than the key descriptors provided on the score sheet. The examiner should refer to the more detailed descriptions of the item for clarification of the weight-bearing, posture, and antigravity movements associated with each item. To receive credit for an item, the infant must exhibit all of the key descriptors noted on the score sheet.

The examiner may place a very young infant in the supine position. The supine subscale has the least number of items because as infants' motor skills mature they do not stay in the supine position for long periods. Rather, they prefer to play in prone, sitting, or standing positions. As a result, the supine items are often not observed in an older infant. The examiner may ask the parent or caregiver to place an infant in the supine position to observe the pattern of rolling, but it is not expected that a series of supine items will be observed spontaneously in an older infant. For an older infant whose motor skills are beyond the supine items, the examiner can place the infant in supine at the end of the assessment and observe the last supine item, *Rolling Supine to Prone with Rotation*. With credit for this item in the motor window the infant can then receive credit for all supine items.

Each item is accompanied by a graph depicting the percentage of infants in the normative sample for each age category that received credit for the particular item. On each graph, the *x*-axis indicates the age in months, and the *y*-axis represents the percentage of infants receiving credit for the item. A solid line has been drawn to indicate the age at which 50% of infants received credit for the item. A dotted line has been drawn at the age at which 90% of infants successfully completed the item. For example, in the *hands to feet* item, 50% of 4.5-month-old infants and 90% of 6-month-old infants successfully performed this item. These graphs provide information on the frequency distribution of the age of attainment of each skill.

Supine Lying (1)

Weight Bearing	Weight on face, side of head, and trunk
Posture	Head rotated to one side Physiological flexion
Antigravity Movement	Head rotation Mouth to hand Random arm and leg movements (stretching)

The infant may move out of the flexed posture but returns to flexion as the resting posture.

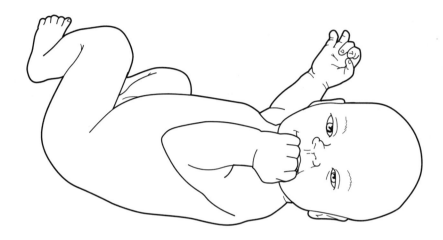

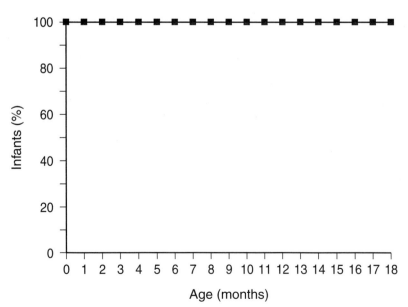

Supine lying (1)

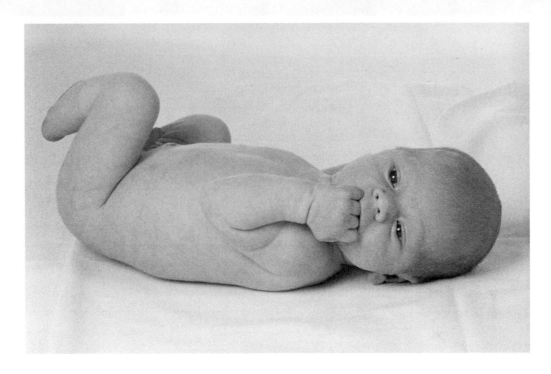

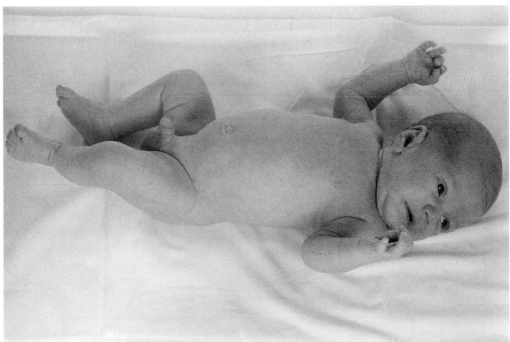

Supine Lying (2)

Weight Bearing	Weight on side of head, trunk, and buttocks
Posture	Physiological flexion diminishing Head rotated to one side Hips abducted and externally rotated Hands open or closed
Antigravity Movement	Head rotation toward midline Random arm and leg movements Nonobligatory asymmetrical tonic neck reflex may be present
The infant may move the head toward midline but cannot maintain the midline position.	
Prompt: May use visual stimulus for head rotation.	

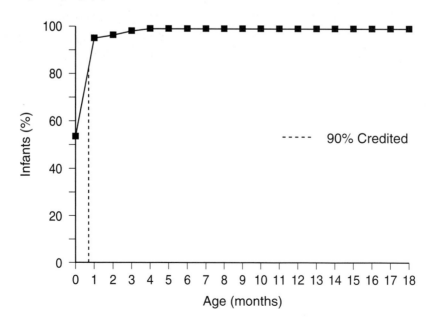

Supine lying (2)

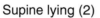

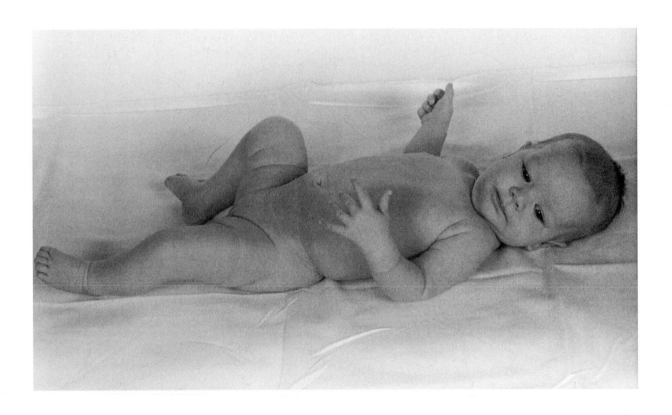

Supine Lying (3)

Weight Bearing	Weight symmetrically distributed on head, trunk, and buttocks
Posture	Head in midline Arms flexed and abducted or positioned at side of body Legs flexed or extended
Antigravity Movement	Bilateral or reciprocal kicking Moves arms but unable to bring hands to midline

The posture of the legs may vary between flexion and extension. The infant is still moving the arms at the side rather than playing in midline.

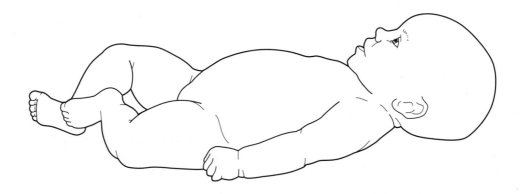

Supine lying (3)

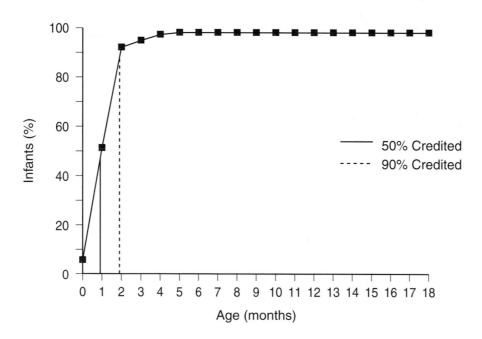

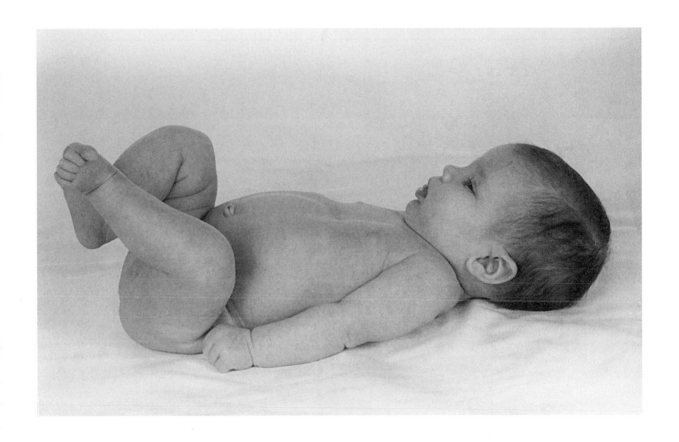

Supine Lying (4)

Weight Bearing	Weight symmetrically distributed on head, trunk, and buttocks
Posture	Head in midline with chin tuck Arms resting on chest Legs flexed or extended
Antigravity Movement	Neck flexors active—chin tuck Brings hands to midline Bilateral or reciprocal kicking

The infant is easily able to bring the hands together in the midline but does not have to successfully grasp a toy to pass this item.

Prompt: May use toy to observe progression of hands to midline.

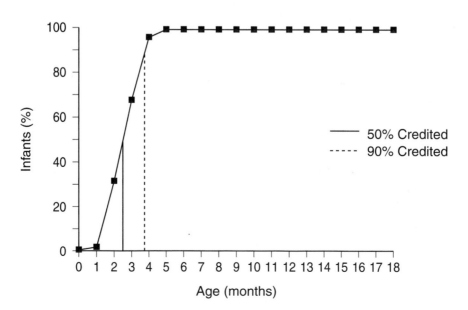

Supine lying (4)

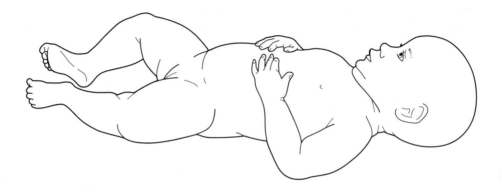

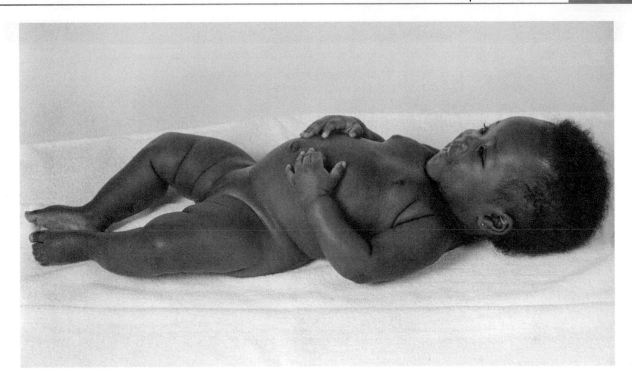

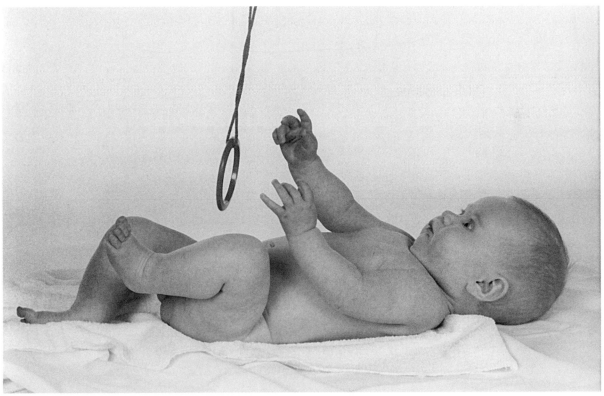

Hands to Knees

Weight Bearing	Weight symmetrically distributed on head, trunk, and pelvis
Posture	Hips abducted and externally rotated Knees flexed
Antigravity Movement	Turns head easily side to side Chin tuck Reaches hand or hands to knees Abdominal muscles active May fall to side by lifting legs

It is important to observe active abdominal muscles. If the legs are widely abducted and resting on the abdomen passively, the infant will not pass this item. Hypotonic infants often display this passive position.

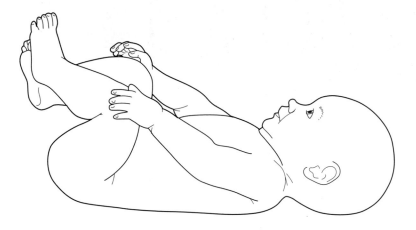

Hands to knees

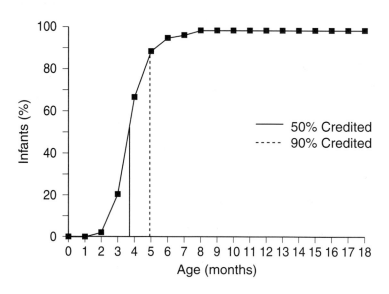

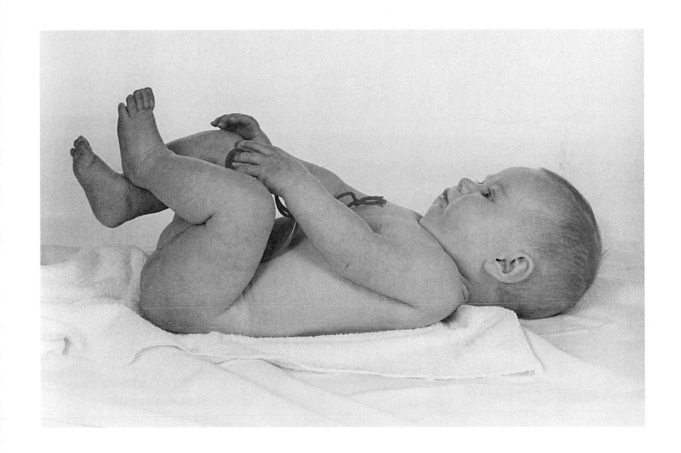

Active Extension	
Weight Bearing	Weight on one side of body
Posture	Hyperextension of neck and spine
Antigravity Movement	Shoulders protracted Pushes into extension with one or both legs May roll to side accidentally

During this movement, one buttock usually remains on the supporting surface. This is a movement that the infant plays with, distinguishing it from the "arching" of hypertonic infants.

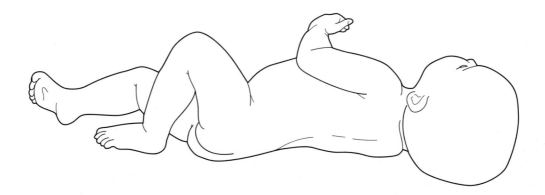

Active extension

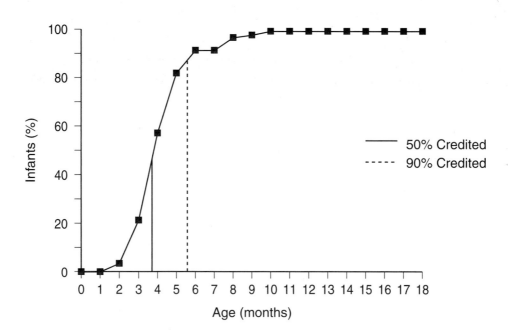

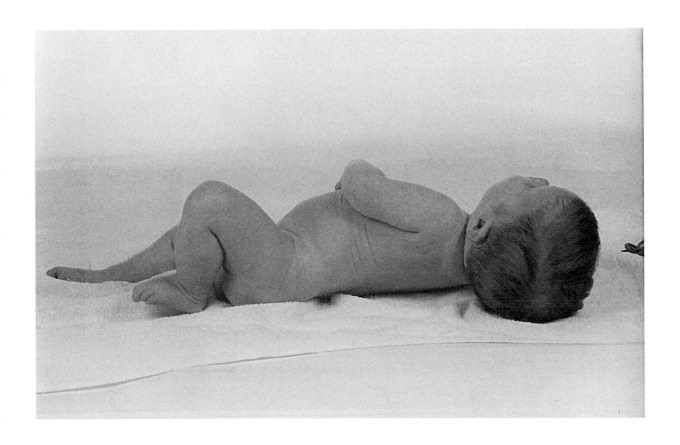

Hands to Feet

Weight Bearing	Weight on head and trunk
Posture	Hand contact with one or both feet Hips flexed greater than 90° Knees semiflexed or extended
Antigravity Movement	Chin tuck Lifts legs and brings feet to hands Can maintain legs in midrange Pelvic mobility present Rocks from side to side; may roll to side

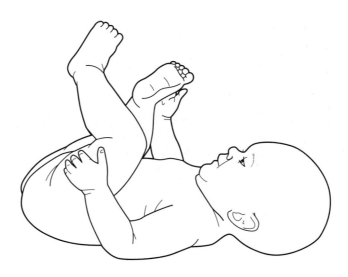

Hands to feet

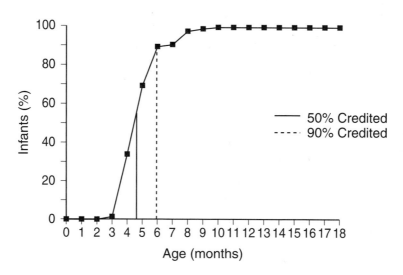

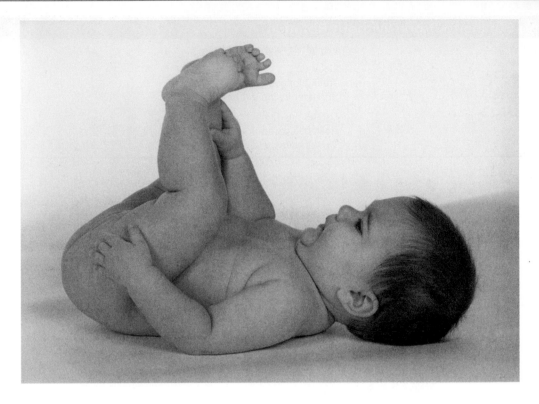

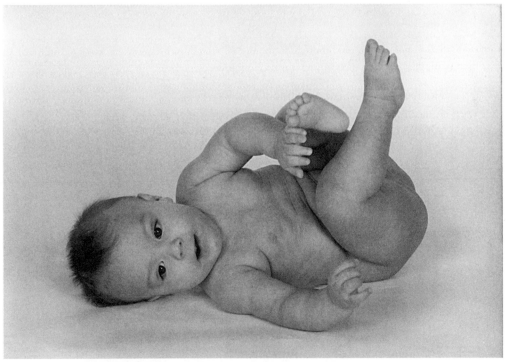

Rolling Supine to Prone Without Rotation

Weight Bearing	Weight on one side of body
Posture	Head up Trunk elongated on weight-bearing side Shoulder in line with pelvis
Antigravity Movement	Lateral head righting Rolling initiated from head, shoulder, or hip Trunk moves as one unit

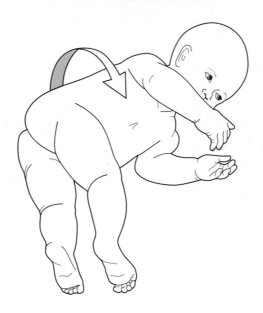

Rolling supine to prone without rotation

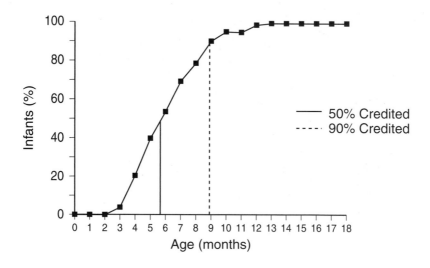

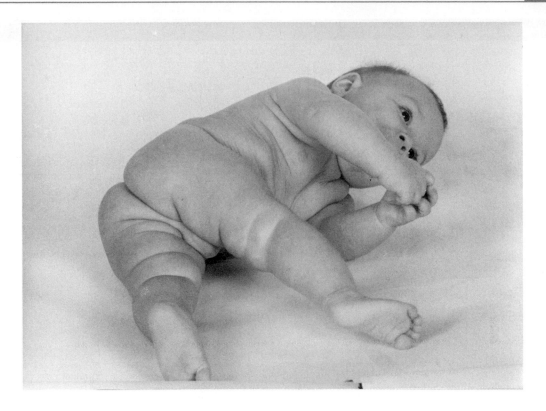

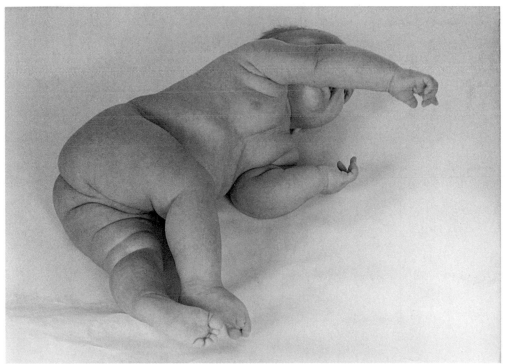

Rolling Supine to Prone With Rotation	
Weight Bearing	Weight on one side of body
Posture	Head up Trunk elongated on weight-bearing side Shoulder and pelvis not aligned
Antigravity Movement	Lateral head righting Dissociated movement in legs Rolling initiated from head, shoulder, or hip Trunk rotation

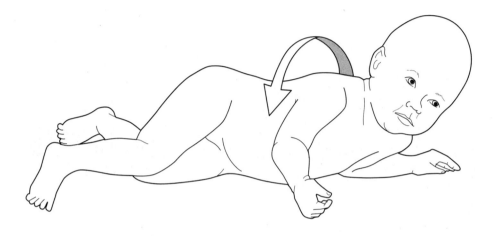

Rolling supine to prone with rotation

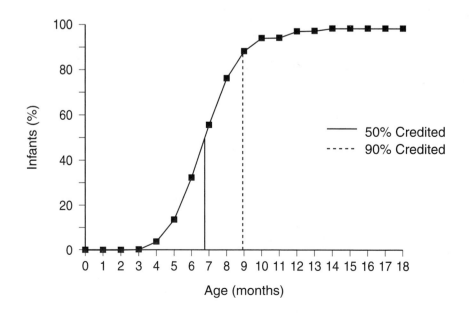

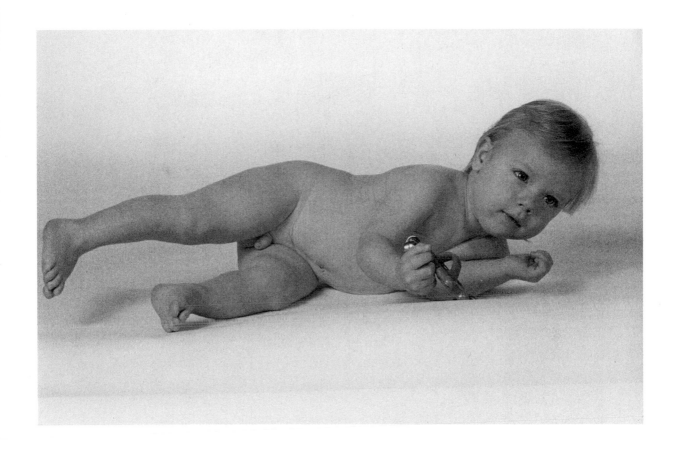

7

Sit Subscale

The sit subscale contains 12 items. Each item consists of an artist's drawing of an infant accompanied by a photograph of a baby performing the movement. A detailed description of the weight-bearing, posture, and antigravity movements observed in each position is included with each item. These descriptions are more detailed than the key descriptors provided on the score sheet. The examiner should refer to the more detailed descriptions of the item for clarification of the weight-bearing, posture, and antigravity movements associated with each item. To receive credit for an item, the infant must exhibit all of the key descriptors noted on the score sheet.

The first item, *sitting with support*, and the third item, *pull to sit,* require physical handling; all other items are observed without assistance from the examiner. Since an infant usually maintains sitting independently before being able to get in and out of the position independently, the examiner can place an infant in the sitting position to observe posture and movements.

Each item is accompanied by a graph depicting the percentage of infants in the normative sample for each age category that received credit for the particular item. On each graph, the *x*-axis indicates the age in months, and the *y*-axis represents the percentage of infants receiving credit for the item. A solid line has been drawn to indicate the age at which 50% of infants received credit for the item. A dotted line has been drawn at the age at which 90% of infants successfully completed the item. For example, in the *unsustained sitting* item, 50% of 4.5-month-old infants and 90% of 6-month-old infants successfully performed this item. These graphs provide information on the frequency distribution of the age of attainment of each skill.

Sitting With Support

Weight Bearing	Weight on buttocks and legs
Posture	Hip flexion Trunk flexion
Antigravity Movement	Lifts and maintains head in midline briefly Upper cervical spine extension

To pass this item, the infant must maintain the head in midline briefly. There must be more head control than "bobbing," but the head does not have to be maintained in midline indefinitely.

Prompt: The infant is supported by examiner around upper trunk.

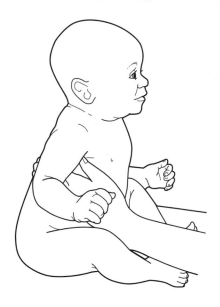

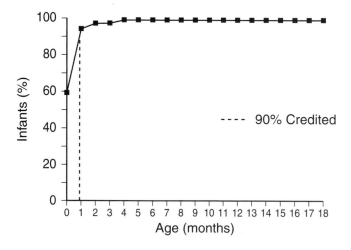

Sitting with support

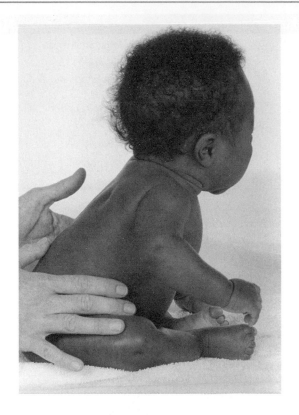

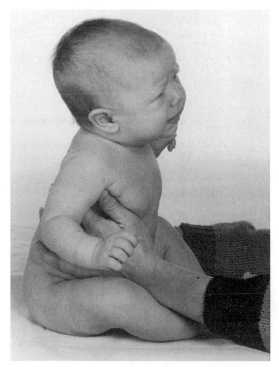

Sitting With Propped Arms

Weight Bearing	Weight on buttocks, legs, and hands
Posture	Head up; shoulders elevated Hips flexed, externally rotated, and abducted Knees flexed Lumbar and thoracic spine rounded
Antigravity Movement	Maintains head in midline Supports weight on arms briefly

Prompt: Examiner places the infant in sitting position. To pass this item, the infant must maintain the position independently without the examiner's support.

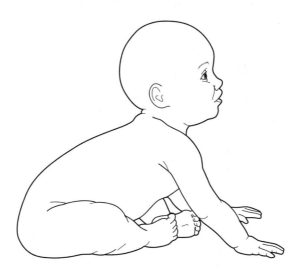

Sitting with propped arms

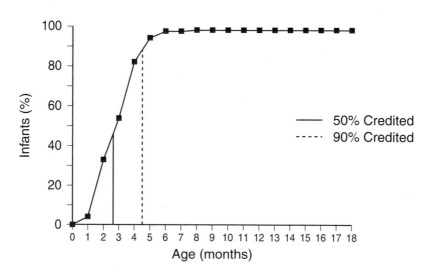

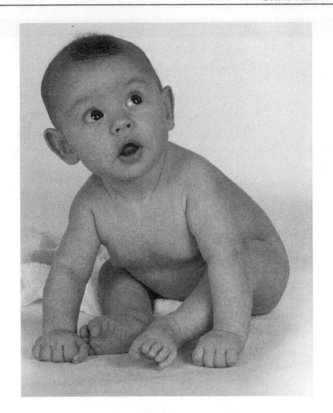

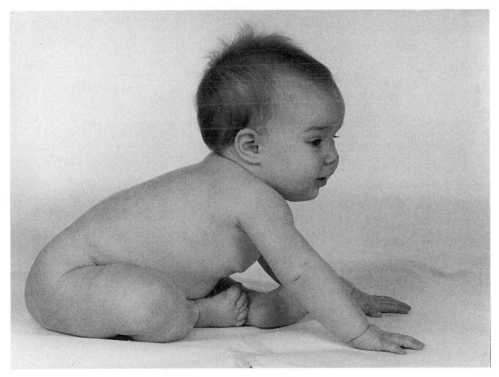

Pull to Sit

Weight Bearing	Weight on buttocks and lumbar spine
Posture	Arms flexed Hips and knees flexed Feet may be off surface
Antigravity Movement	Chin tucked; head in line or in front of body May assist movement with abdominal muscles and arm flexion

At the initiation of the movement, there may be a slight head lag, which the infant quickly overcomes. There may be varying degrees of flexion in the legs as the infant assists with the movement.

Prompt. Examiner pulls infant to sit by holding the wrists.

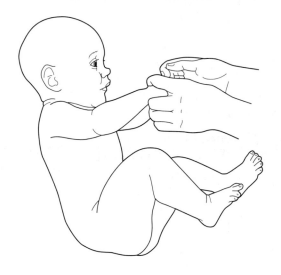

Pull to sit

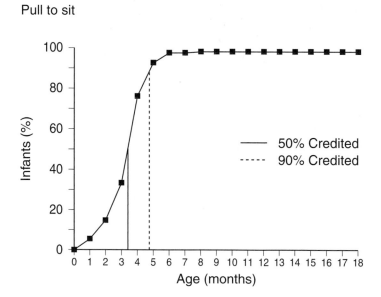

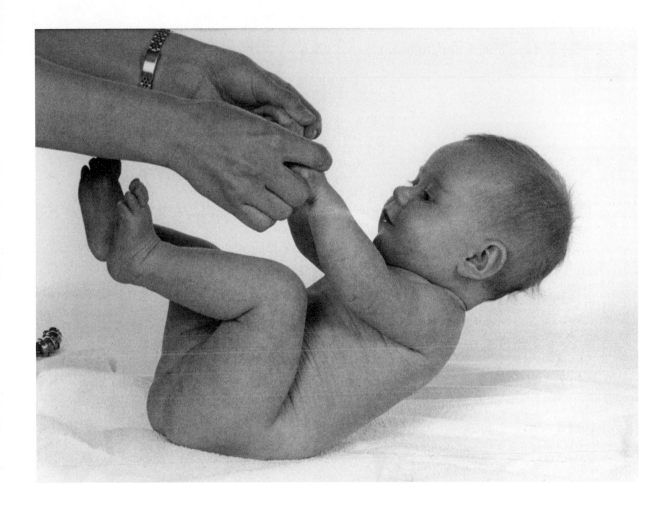

Unsustained Sitting

Weight Bearing	Weight on buttocks and legs
Posture	Head in midline Shoulders in front of hips Thoracic spine extended Lumbar flexion Hips flexed and externally rotated
Antigravity Movement	Head extension Scapular adduction and humeral extension Cannot maintain position indefinitely

Prompt: Examiner places infant in sitting position. To pass this item, the infant must maintain the position briefly and not fall over immediately.

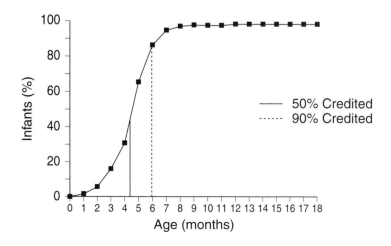

Unsustained sitting

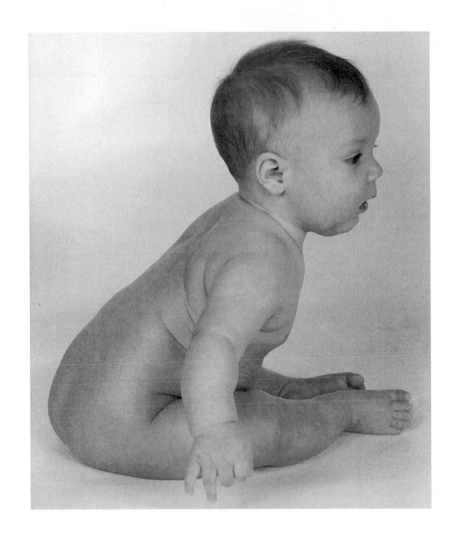

Sitting With Arm Support

Weight Bearing	Weight on buttocks, legs, and hands
Posture	Head up Lumbar spine rounded, thoracic spine extended Extended arm support Hips flexed, externally rotated, and abducted Knees flexed
Antigravity Movement	Head movements free from trunk Propped on extended arms Cannot move in and out of position
Prompt: Examiner places the infant in sitting position.	

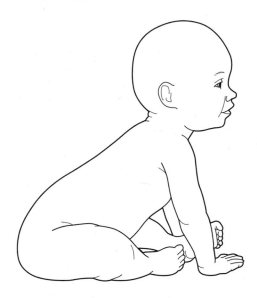

Sitting with arm support

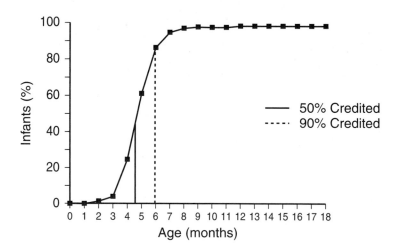

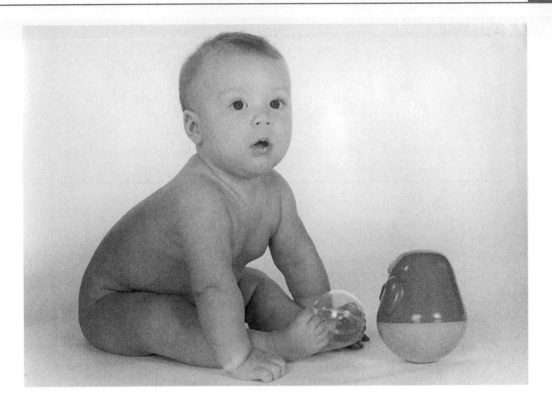

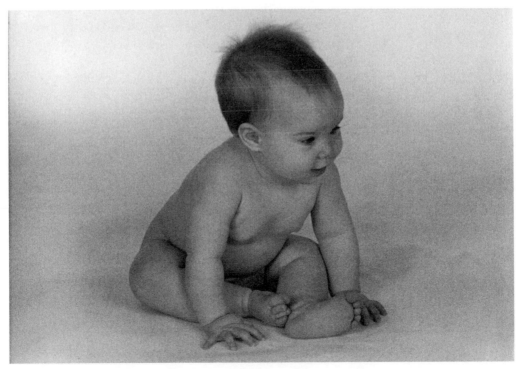

Unsustained Sitting Without Arm Support

Weight Bearing	Weight on buttocks and legs
Posture	Elbows flexed Thoracic spine extended Hips flexed, externally rotated, and abducted with wide base of support Knees flexed
Antigravity Movement	Cannot be left alone in sitting position indefinitely
To pass this item, the infant must be able to maintain sitting alone for a brief period but still may require supervision.	
Prompt: Examiner places the infant in sitting position.	

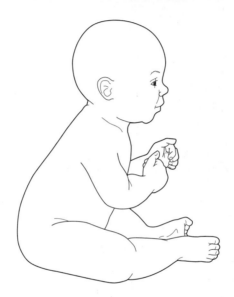

Unsustained sitting without arm support

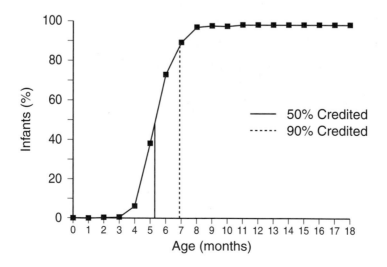

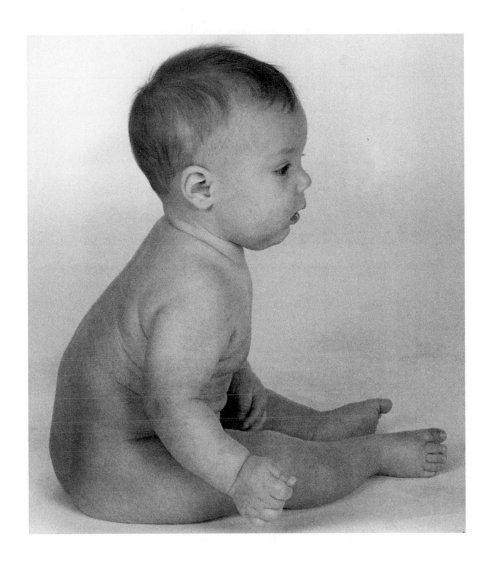

Weight Shift in Unsustained Sitting

Weight Bearing	Weight on buttocks and legs
Posture	Hips flexed, abducted, and externally rotated Arms free
Antigravity Movement	Weight shift forward, backward, or sideways Beginning to right body back to midline Cannot be left alone in sitting position

This item represents a stage in sitting in which an infant loses balance easily, especially when experimenting with weight shift.

Prompt: Examiner places the infant in sitting position. May use toys to elicit weight shift.

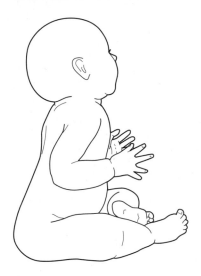

Weight shift in unsustained sitting

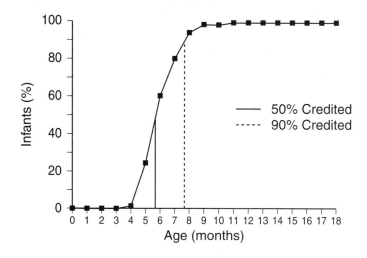

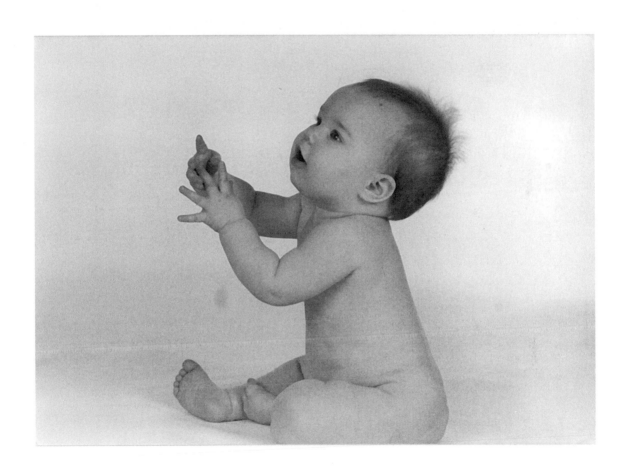

Sitting Without Arm Support (1)

Weight Bearing	Weight on buttocks and legs
Posture	Shoulders aligned over hips Arms free Wide base of support
Antigravity Movement	Arms move away from body Can play with a toy Can be left alone in sitting position

To pass this item, an infant must be able to maintain sitting well. The caregiver is comfortable leaving the infant in sitting position. Rotation within the trunk does not need to be present to pass this item.

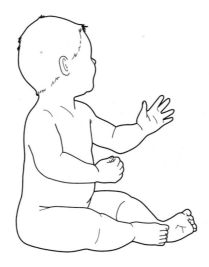

Sitting without arm support (1)

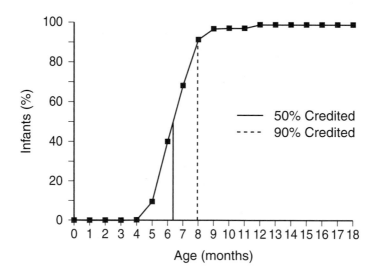

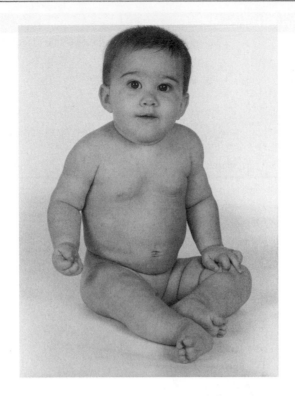

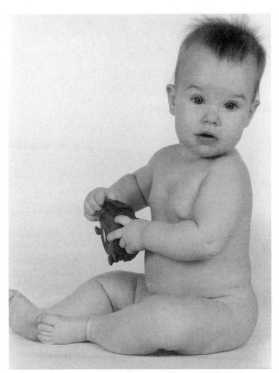

Reach With Rotation in Sitting

Weight Bearing	Weight on buttocks and legs
Posture	Trunk rotated Elongation of trunk on reaching side
Antigravity Movement	Sits independently Reaches for toy with trunk rotation

To pass this item, an infant must be able to easily reach for a toy, and rotation must be seen within the trunk. The infant may reach in any direction as long as trunk rotation is observed.

Prompt. Examiner may place infant in sitting position. May use toys to encourage infant to reach.

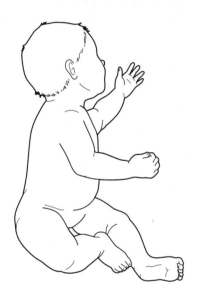

Reach with rotation in sitting

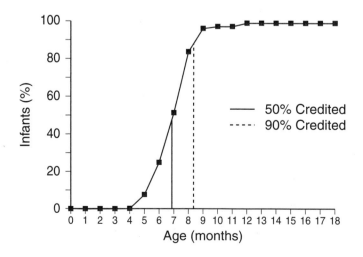

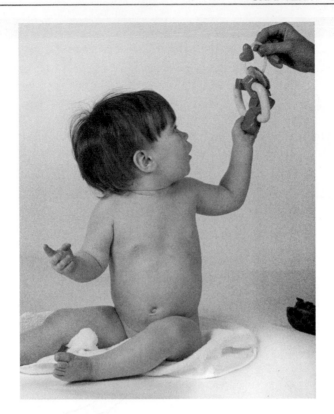

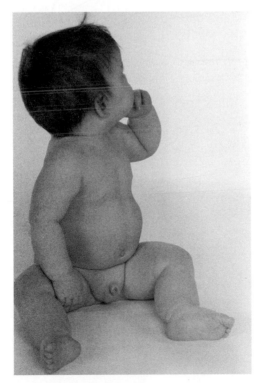

Sitting to Prone

Weight Bearing	Weight on hands, forearms, and trunk
Posture	Trunk flexed anteriorly or sideways over lower extremities Legs flexed, abducted, and externally rotated
Antigravity Movement	Moves out of sitting position to achieve prone lying position Pulls with arms; legs inactive

To pass this item, the infant must be able to maintain sitting with or without arm support. The infant may or may not use trunk rotation to get to prone position. This item is often observed as the infant's first attempt to move out of sitting position. The item can be passed even if it is performed in an immature manner.

Prompt. Examiner may place the infant in sitting position.

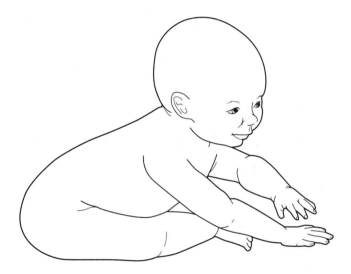

Sitting to prone

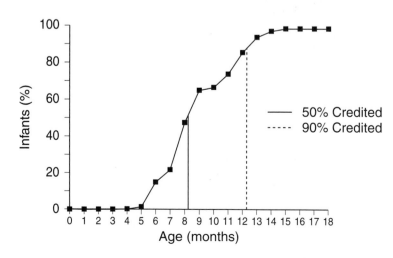

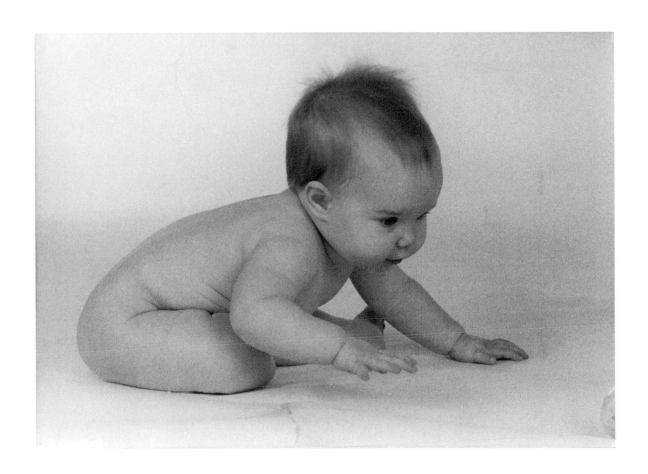

Sitting to Four-Point Kneeling

Weight Bearing	Weight on both hands and one foot
Posture	Moves from an independent sitting position to four-point kneeling
Antigravity Movement	Actively lifts pelvis, buttocks, and unweighted leg to assume four-point kneeling position

To pass this item the infant must be able to maintain sitting without arm support. A variety of ways may be demonstrated to assume four-point kneeling; the critical element is that it is a controlled movement and the pelvis is elevated—the infant cannot "flop" into prone position.

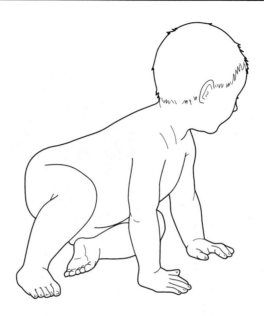

Sitting to four-point kneeling

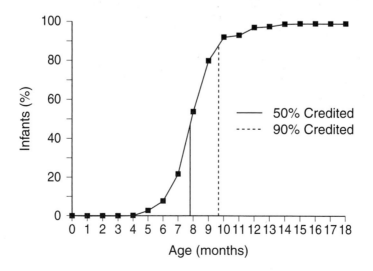

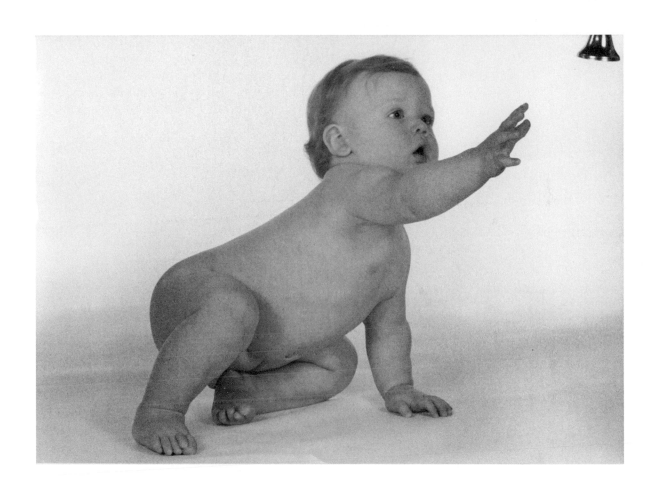

Sitting Without Arm Support (2)

Weight Bearing	Weight on buttocks
Posture	Variety of postures with dissociation of legs Narrow base of support
Antigravity Movement	Position of legs varies Infant moves in and out of positions easily

This item can be passed if a variety of sitting postures are observed; these include "W" sitting and side sitting. It is important to ascertain that the infant has more than one sitting posture in the movement repertoire. The infant must assume the position independently.

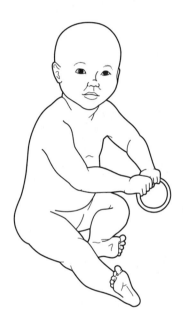

Sitting without arm support (2)

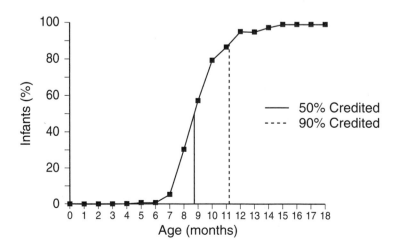

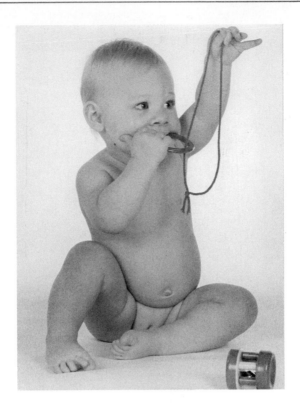

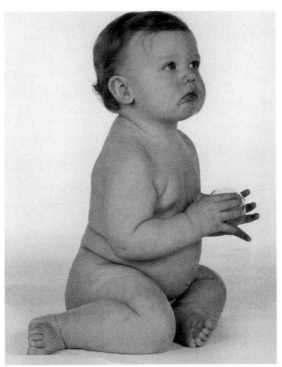

8

Stand Subscale

The stand subscale contains 16 items. Each item consists of an artist's drawing of an infant accompanied by a photograph of a baby performing the movement. A detailed description of the weight-bearing, posture, and antigravity movements observed in each position is included with each item. These descriptions are more detailed than the key descriptors provided on the score sheet. The examiner should refer to the more detailed descriptors of the item for clarification of the weight-bearing, posture, and antigravity movements associated with each item. To receive credit for an item, the infant must exhibit all of the key descriptors noted on the score sheet.

To observe the first three standing items, the examiner must support the infant in a standing position. To receive credit for any of the remaining items in the stand subscale, the infant must assume standing independently.

Each item is accompanied by a graph depicting the percentage of infants in the normative sample for each age category that received credit for the particular item. On each graph, the x-axis indicates the age in months, and the y-axis represents the percentage of infants receiving credit for the item. A solid line has been drawn to indicate the age at which 50% of infants received credit for the item. A dotted line has been drawn at the age at which 90% of infants successfully completed the item. For example, in the *stands alone* item, 50% of 10.5-month-old infants and 90% of 13-month-old infants successfully performed this item. These graphs provide information on the frequency distribution of the age of attainment of each skill.

Supported Standing (1)	
Weight Bearing	Bears weight intermittently
Posture	Head flexed forward Hips behind shoulders Hips and knees flexed Feet may be close together Infant does not slip through examiner's hands
Antigravity Movement	There may be intermittent hip and knee flexion
Prompt: Supported by examiner under axillae.	

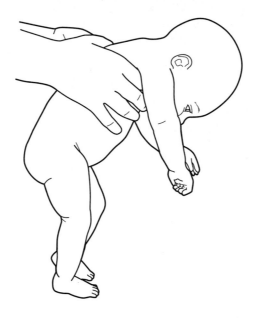

Supported standing (1)

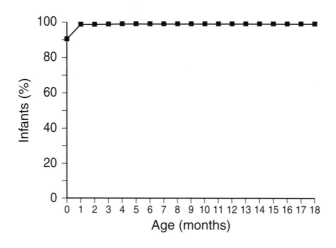

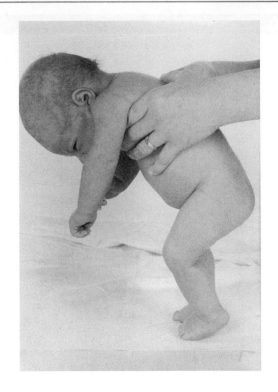

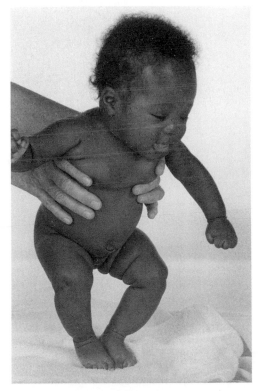

Supported Standing (2)	
Weight Bearing	Weight on feet or toes
Posture	Head in line with body Hips behind shoulders Hips flexed and abducted
Antigravity Movement	Variable movement of legs May bend and straighten knees May hyperextend knees May stamp with one foot

The antigravity movements observed in the legs are extremely variable. Some flexion of the legs is observed in the resting posture.

Prompt: The infant is supported by examiner under the axillae.

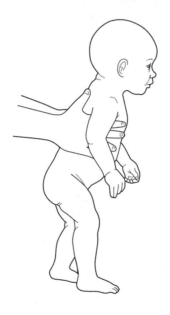

Supported standing (2)

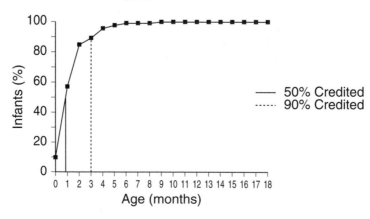

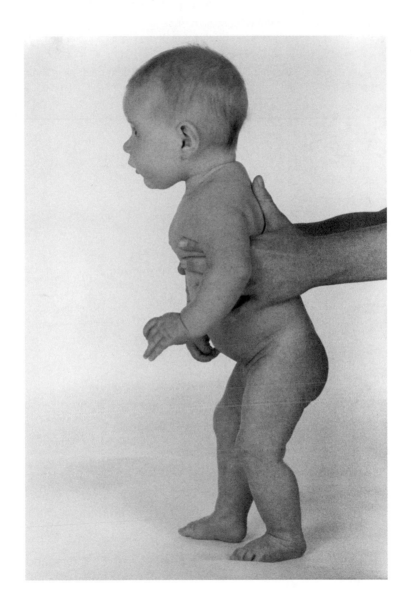

Supported Standing (3)	
Weight Bearing	Weight on feet
Posture	Head in midline Hips in line with shoulders Hips abducted and externally rotated
Antigravity Movement	Active control of trunk Variable movements of legs: may bounce up and down, lift one leg, or hyperextend the knees
The antigravity movements are extremely variable. To pass this item, the infant must have the heels down at some point during the observation period and demonstrate spontaneous movement in the legs.	
Prompt: Infant is supported by examiner at chest level.	

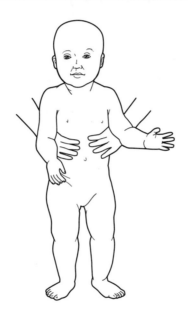

Supported standing (3)

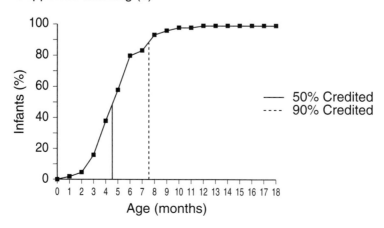

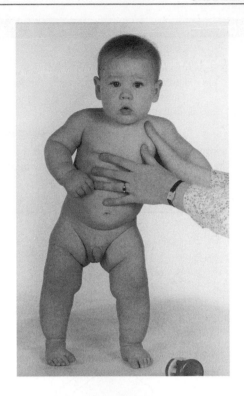

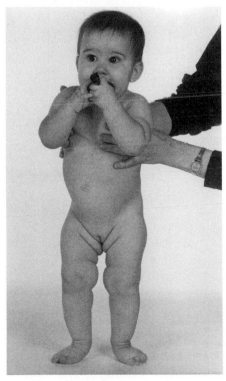

Pulls to Stand With Support

Weight Bearing	Weight on arms and feet
Posture	Arms on support Hips abducted and externally rotated Leans on support Lumbar lordosis
Antigravity Movement	Pushes down with arms and extends knees to achieve standing

The legs do not have to be completely symmetrical during this maneuver, and the infant may push with the legs to assume the position. The posture of the feet is variable; weight bearing may be observed on the toes or medial border of the feet.

Prompt: May use toys to encourage infant to get to standing position. Do not place in standing position.

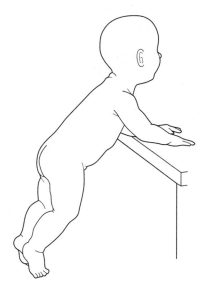

Pulls to stand with support

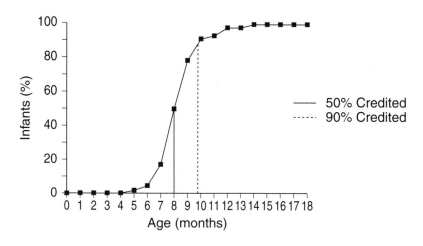

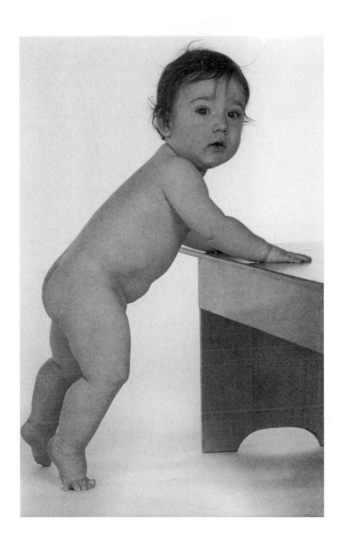

Pulls to Stand/Stands

Weight Bearing	Weight on feet Some arm support
Posture	Hips flexed, abducted, and externally rotated Lumbar lordosis Broad stance
Antigravity Movement	Pulls to stand Shifts weight from side to side May lift one leg off surface No rotation in trunk

The examiner must observe the infant independently assume the standing position. The infant may pull to stand through postures other than half-kneeling.

Prompt: May use toys to encourage infant to stand.

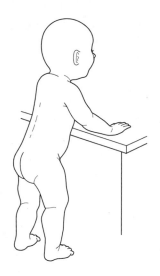

Pulls to stand/stands

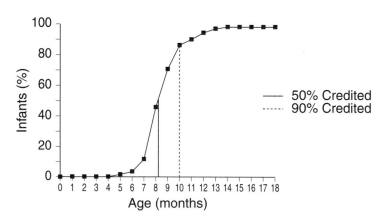

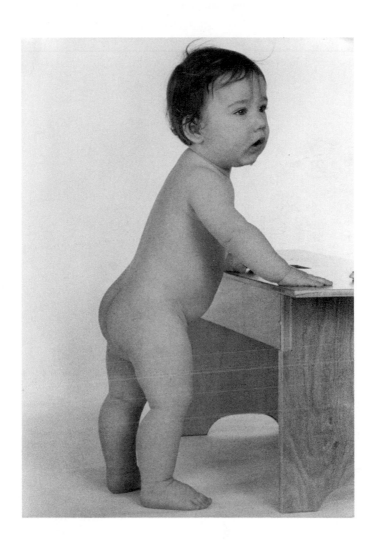

Supported Standing With Rotation

Weight Bearing	Weight on feet One-arm support
Posture	Hips abducted Trunk rotated
Antigravity Movement	Able to release one hand and reach with rotation of trunk and pelvis

If the infant is not observed to pull to stand independently, he or she should not pass this item. The infant's base of support may still be wide.

Prompt: May use toys to elicit trunk rotation.

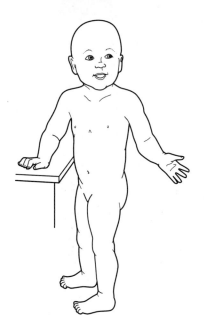

Supported standing with rotation

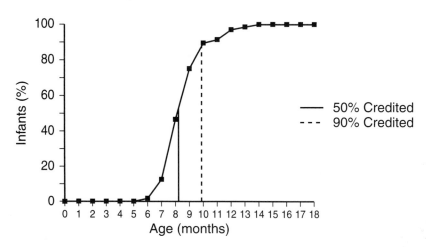

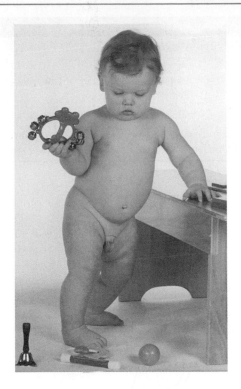

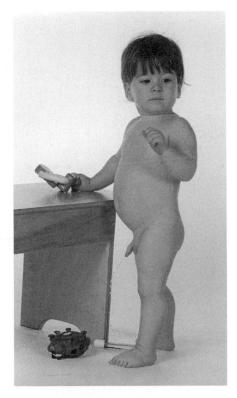

Cruising Without Rotation

Weight Bearing	Weight on feet Some arm support
Posture	Legs abducted and externally rotated Wide base of support
Antigravity Movement	Cruises sideways without rotation

If the infant is not observed to pull to stand independently, he or she should not pass this item. The infant may go up on the toes in standing but should be observed to assume a plantigrade position some of the time.

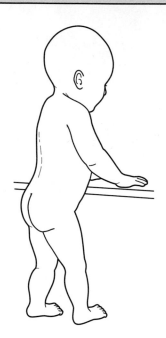

Cruising without rotation

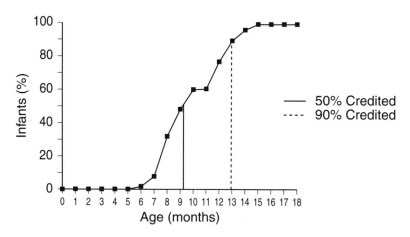

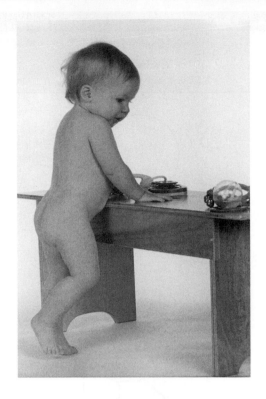

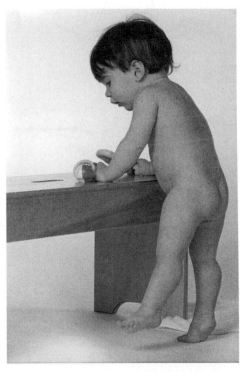

Half-Kneeling

Weight Bearing	Weight on one flexed knee and the opposite foot; arm support
Posture	Half-kneeling posture
Antigravity Movement	May assume standing or play in position

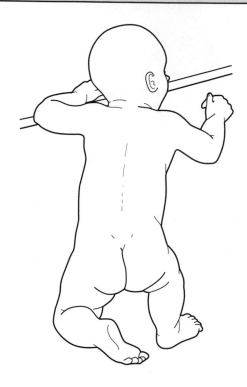

Half-kneeling

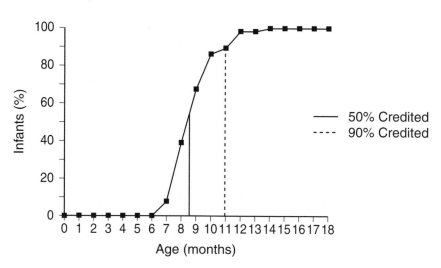

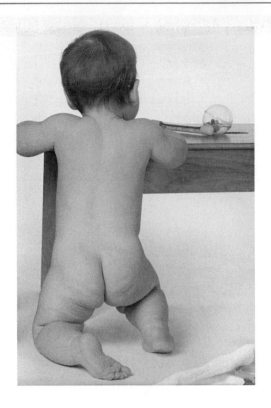

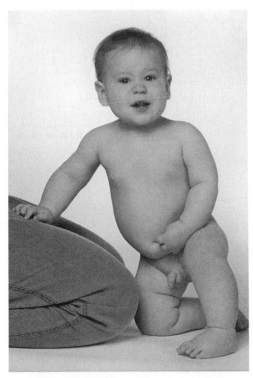

Controlled Lowering From Standing

Weight Bearing	Weight on feet
	One-arm support
Posture	Holds onto support with one hand
Antigravity Movement	Controlled lowering from standing

To pass this item, the infant must assume standing independently. A variety of leg postures may be observed; the legs may move symmetrically or asymmetrically. The movement must be controlled, and the infant must not accidentally fall from the standing position. The infant does not have to return to standing.

Prompt: May use toys to elicit the antigravity movements.

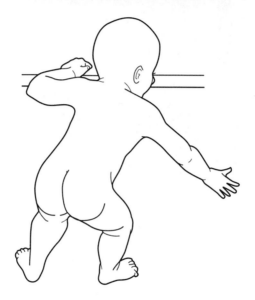

Controlled lowering from standing

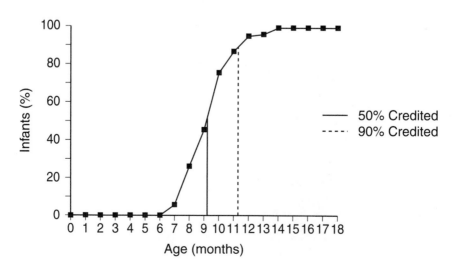

50% Credited
90% Credited

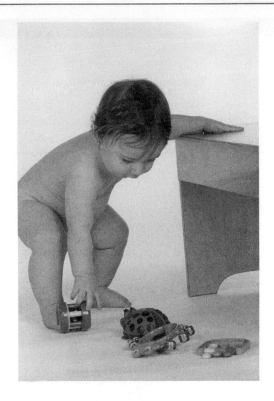

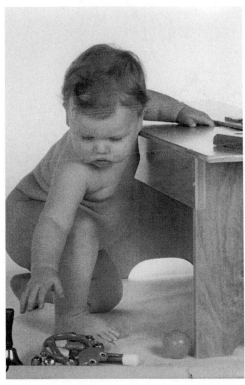

Cruising With Rotation

Weight Bearing	Weight on feet Some arm support
Posture	Semiturned in direction of movement
Antigravity Movement	Cruises with rotation
If the infant is not observed to pull to stand independently, he or she should not pass this item.	
Prompt: May use toys to encourage infant to cruise.	

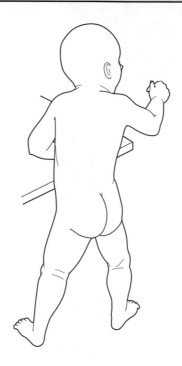

Cruising with rotation

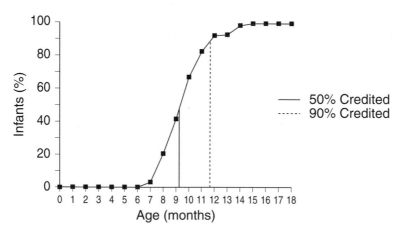

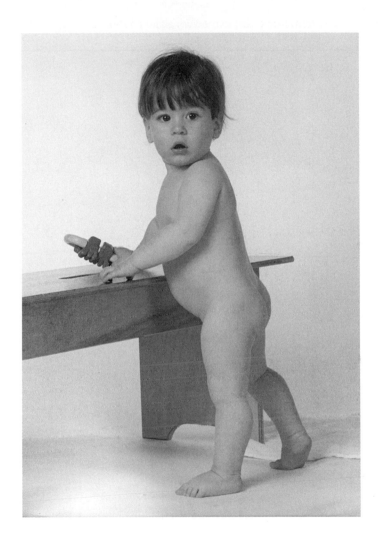

Stands Alone

Weight Bearing	Weight on feet
Posture	Scapular adduction Lumbar lordosis Hips abducted and externally rotated
Antigravity Movement	Stands alone momentarily Balance reactions in feet

The position of the arms may vary from high guard to medium guard position. Balance reactions in the feet can be either dorsiflexion balance reactions or intermittent toe grasping.

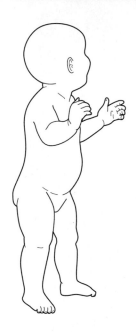

Stands alone

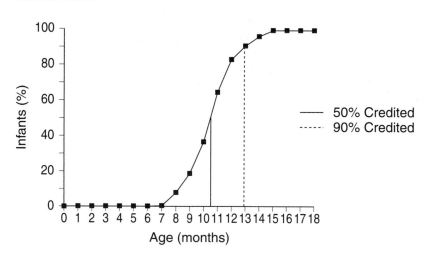

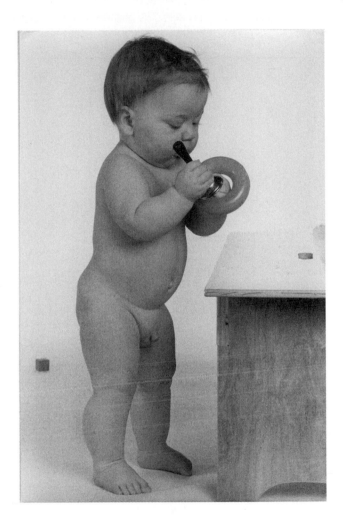

Early Stepping

Weight Bearing	Weight on feet
Posture	Scapular adduction Lumbar lordosis Legs abducted and externally rotated
Antigravity Movement	Walks independently Moves quickly with short steps

The infant must take five independent steps to pass this item. The position of the arms may vary from high guard to medium guard position. This item represents the infant's first attempts to walk independently; he or she may still fall often.

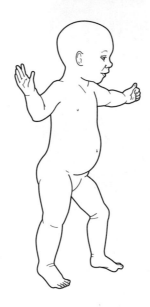

Early stepping

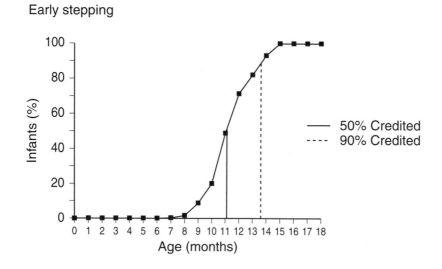

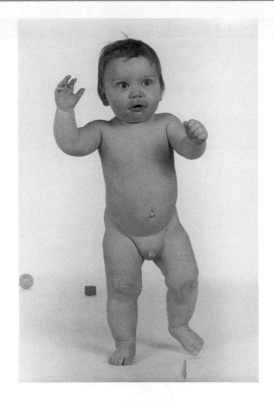

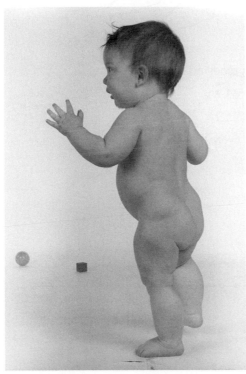

Standing From Modified Squat

Weight Bearing	Weight on feet
Posture	Squat position
Antigravity Movement	Moves from standing to squat and back to standing with controlled flexion and extension of hips and knees

To pass this item, the infant does not have to maintain the squat position; he or she may quickly move from squat position back to standing.

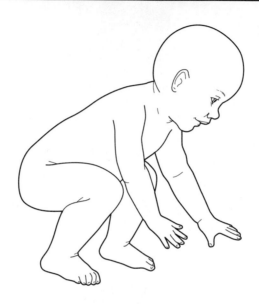

Standing from modified squat

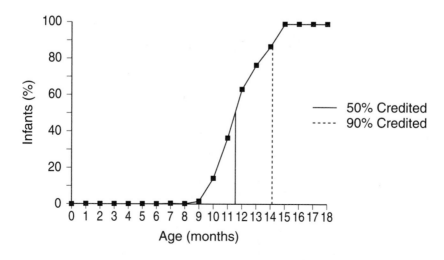

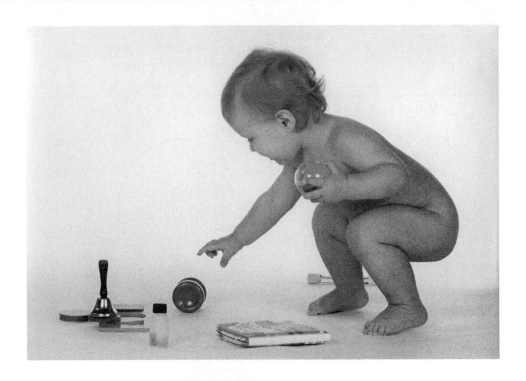

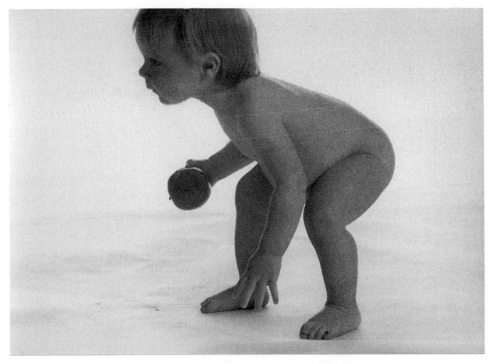

Standing From Quadruped Position

Weight Bearing	Weight on hands and feet
Posture	Hands and feet
Antigravity Movement	Assumes standing independently Pushes quickly with hands to get to standing without using any props

Prompt: To elicit this item, the examiner may position the infant in the supine position and observe the response.

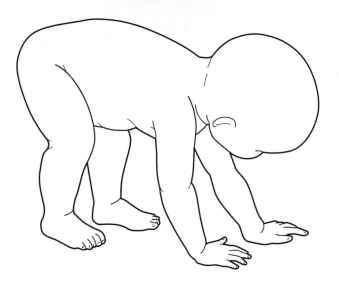

Standing from quadruped position

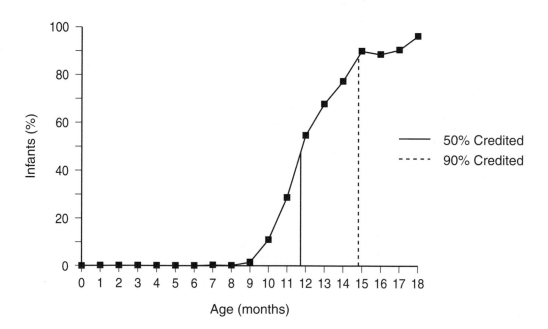

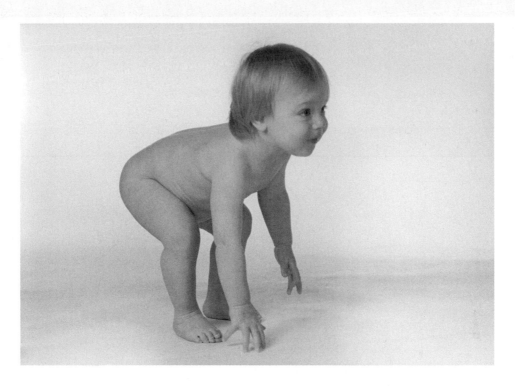

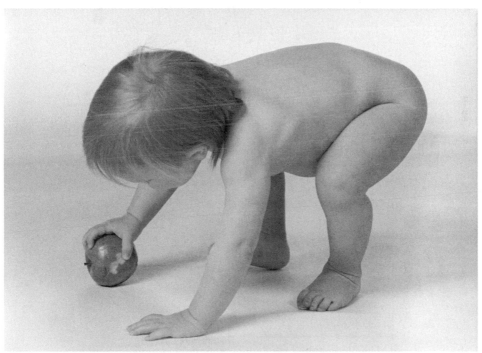

Walks Alone

Weight Bearing	Weight on feet
Posture	Arms may vary from medium guard to low guard to side of body positions Lumbar lordosis Legs neutral or slightly abducted
Antigravity Movement	Walks independently

To pass this item, the infant uses walking as the main method of locomotion. The walking pattern may still be immature.

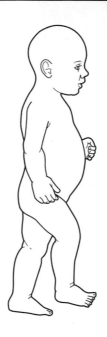

Walks alone

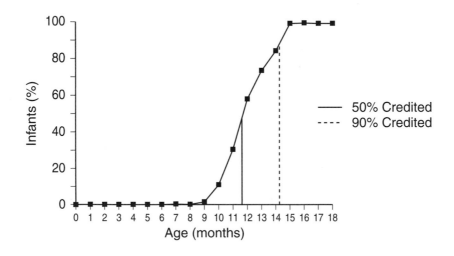

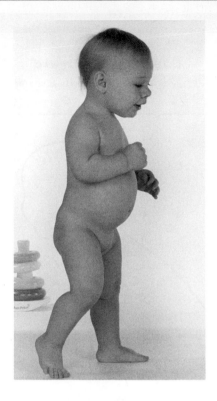

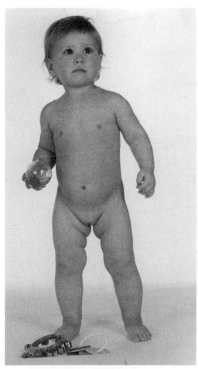

Squat	
Weight Bearing	Weight on feet
Posture	Squat posture; trunk forward
Antigravity Movement	Maintains position by balance reactions in feet and position of trunk
The infant is able to play in this position.	

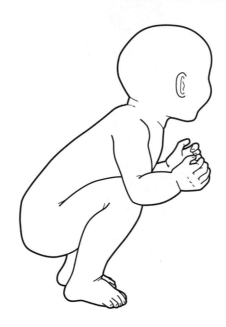

Squat

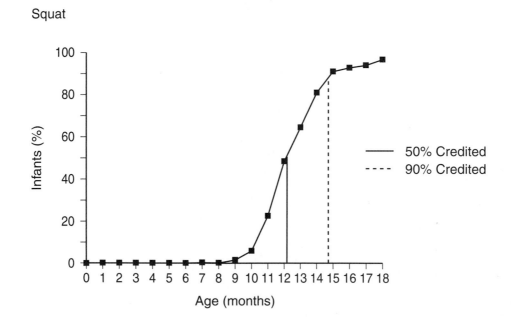

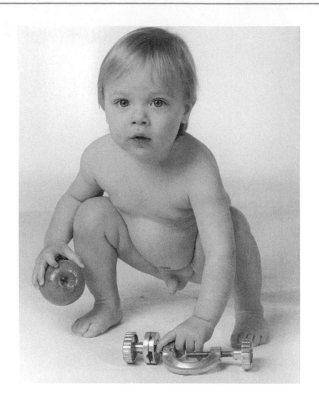

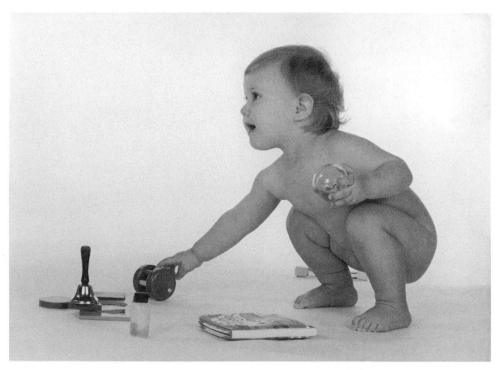

Clinical Uses of the Alberta Infant Motor Scale

Which test to use with whom, when, and for what purpose? Clinicians face this dilemma when choosing a measure to assess the gross motor development of infants at risk for neuromotor delays. An array of infant assessment tools is available to describe and to record infant gross motor abilities. When selecting a clinical measure to use for an infant assessment, factors such as the psychometric properties of the test, the age group for which the test was developed, and the time needed for administration and scoring need to be considered (Spittle et al., 2008). The primary purpose of the measure should be clearly stated. A discriminative or identification measure provides information about an infant's present performance compared to a normative comparative group. An evaluative measure captures changes in performance over time, while a predictive measure is used to determine the eventual motor outcome of an infant. A diagnostic measure establishes the presence of a specific condition. This chapter provides an overview of the appropriate use of the Alberta Infant Motor Scale (AIMS), including a description of the type of infants that can be assessed for each of these purposes.

DISCRIMINATION (IDENTIFICATION)

The primary purpose of the AIMS is discrimination; it may be used to compare an infant's current gross motor performance to an age-matched normative group from birth to 18 months of age. The normative data, presented in weekly age intervals, provide information regarding an infant's score compared to other infants in the same age interval. For example, an infant whose total score falls below the 5th percentile rank for that age group has a score that is lower than 95% of the infants of the same age in the normative sample. The robust psychometric properties of the AIMS and the large normative sample make it a strong discriminative index of infant gross motor maturity.

As a discriminative index the AIMS may be used to assess the gross motor maturity of all infants from birth to 18 months of life. Clinicians may use an AIMS score as one component of the information they use in making clinical decisions regarding an infant's motor performance. Other sources of information, including the infant's medical history, a full clinical examination, and parents' concerns, need to be considered. The interpretation of gross motor information from an AIMS assessment requires professional judgment that takes into consideration the age of the infant, the infant's history, the severity of the delay, and movement patterns observed. The clinical actions that might be taken as a result of an identified delay in motor development include ongoing monitoring and follow-up, intervention, or more detailed diagnostic testing. Caution is advised in interpreting a single low percentile ranking obtained by an infant as evidence of future motor delay; typically developing infants have demonstrated fluctuations in their AIMS scores from birth to independent walking (Darrah et al., 1998b).

Discrimination

Amy is 4 months old (corrected age). She was born at 28 weeks of gestation and was discharged from hospital at 1 week corrected age still requiring oxygen. She has been referred for a physical therapy assessment because of parent concerns. Her AIMS score falls below the 5th percentile rank for her age group, suggesting that her gross motor skills are lower than 95% of infants of the same age in the normative sample. Follow-up by the physical therapist and intervention suggestions are recommended.

EVALUATION

The AIMS may be used to identify changes in the motor abilities of infants 18 months old or younger who have either typical gross motor skills or who have delayed, immature gross motor abilities. AIMS items in each sub-scale capture not only the acquisition of new gross motor skills, but also maturational changes of individual motor skills. For example, in the *prone subscale,* infants will receive additional scoring credit if the pattern of their four-point kneeling changes from an immature, wide-based stance *(Four-Point Kneeling 1)* to a more mature posture with hips aligned under the pelvis and no lumbar lordosis *(Four-Point Kneeling 2).* Infant gross motor tests such as the Peabody Gross and Fine Motor Scales (Folio & Fewell, 2000) evaluate maturational changes within a specific skill by using time and distance as indicators of improvement. The AIMS documents maturational change of a motor skill by describing the components of the skill that may be observed. By using the item descriptors, maturational changes may be evaluated.

Examination of test-retest reliability during the development of the AIMS (see Chapter 10) revealed a one item mean score difference of infants' scores over a 1-week interval suggesting that the AIMS is able to document small changes in an infant's performance. When used to evaluate the effects of intervention with an individual infant, it is not possible to determine if the change score is due to intervention or maturation. Further investigation with large samples sizes is needed to understand how much change in AIMS scores over time represents a clinically important difference in an infant's motor abilities.

The AIMS should not be used to evaluate change in the gross motor skills of children older than 18 months whose motor abilities are at an infant level, or infants and children of any age who use atypical compensatory movement solutions to explore their environment. The normative data cannot be used to derive a percentile rank for infants older than 18 months even though the AIMS items may capture the infant's current motor skills.

Infants younger than 18 months who have discovered innovative but atypical movement solutions should not be evaluated over time using the AIMS items. While they may increase their motor function, this improvement will not be reflected in their AIMS scores since they move in a way that does not meet the criteria of the descriptors on the AIMS items. For example, infants with a diagnosis of spastic diplegia may learn to explore their environment by using a symmetrical movement of their arms and legs with their legs flexed and their arms extended rather than using typical creeping as described in *Reciprocal Creeping (1)* and *Reciprocal Creeping (2).* Despite having improved their independence and ability to explore their environment, they will not receive credit for the functional improvement in their mobility on the AIMS because they do not demonstrate the specific criteria associated with the two creeping items.

Discrimination and Evaluation

Amy is reassessed at 6 months (corrected age). Her AIMS score is now at the 50th percentile rank for her age group. Her parents are informed that her score has improved for her gross motor skills since her previous assessment (evaluation). The change may be due to neurological maturation, the intervention program, or both. Her gross motor AIMS score is now higher than 50% of infants the same age in the normative sample (discrimination).

PREDICTION AND DIAGNOSIS

The ability of the AIMS to predict the eventual gross motor performance of at-risk infants requires further evaluation. The initial psychometric evaluation of the predictive abilities of the AIMS is described in Chapter 10. Two cutoff points, the 10th percentile at 4 months and the 5th percentile at 8 months, provided the best compromise between sensitivity and specificity values for prediction of motor outcome at 18 months of age (Darrah et al., 1998a). The scores of infants classified as "suspicious" in their motor development at 18 months exhibited lowered sensitivity values when placed in either "normal" or "abnormal" final outcome categories. Examination of this group's scoring distribution revealed a range of scores (0–75th percentile at 4 months and 0–35th percentile at 8 months), suggesting a wide range of motor abilities. A systematic review of five studies that evaluated the ability of the AIMS to predict delayed motor development in preterm infants reported a high risk of study design bias and recommended further evaluation of the AIMS predictive abilities (Albuquerque et al., 2015). Recommendations to improve the clinical prediction of future motor outcome of at-risk infants include serial assessments rather than a single assessment and the use of more than one type of assessment measure (Spittle et al., 2015). If the AIMS is used to predict infants' future motor abilities in conjunction with other measures, the cutoff points of the 10th percentile at 4 month of age and younger and the 5th percentile at 8 months of age and older are recommended. Higher cutoff points will provide improved sensitivity but at the cost of incorrectly identifying typically developing infants as suspicious or delayed (false positives).

Prediction of at-risk infants' eventual gross motor performance developmental outcome is not a perfect science (Aylward, 2009). Theoretical issues and study designs challenge the success of the predictive ability of motor assessments. Contemporary theories of motor development suggest that motor skills are acquired in a variable and nonlinear manner, and thus a low score on one assessment may not represent a true delay but rather a latent period of acquisition of motor skills. Evaluation of the longitudinal motor trajectories of typically developing infants and preschoolers support this theoretical tenet; the majority of children demonstrated fluctuating percentile ranks scores over monthly assessments (Darrah et al., 2009). Published studies evaluating the predictive validity of the AIMS use differing criteria for important variables such as the age of the infants at the initial assessment, the risk status of the infants, and the length of time between the initial assessment and the final outcome, making comparison between studies difficult.

The AIMS should not be used as a diagnostic test. While it provides information regarding the gross motor status of an infant, it does not identify either the reasons or cause of the delay. Information from an AIMS assessment can suggest the presence of immature or atypical movements, but further diagnostic testing is recommended to determine why an infant is using these movement solutions.

Prediction

Amy is assessed at 8 months (corrected age) as part of a preterm follow-up clinic. Her AIMS score continues to be at the 50th percentile for her age group, confirming that she is performing well in her age group (discrimination). Her parents are told that her gross motor skills continue to score within a typical range, and she has a low risk of future gross motor delay (prediction).

PLANNING

The AIMS item descriptors may be useful to therapists when planning an intervention strategy for infants demonstrating immature but typical patterns of movement. Each AIMS item is described according to three components: (1) the part of the body that bears weight, (2) the posture of the infant, and (3) the antigravity movements an infant must demonstrate to receive credit for the item. These descriptors provide a guideline regarding the components of a motor skill necessary for an infant to successfully accomplish the item. Knowledge of the missing components of a specific motor skill may assist a therapist designing an intervention program to encourage an infant to experience the missing components of a specific motor skill. This feature of the AIMS may be especially valuable to therapists who are less experienced and who have not had the opportunity to observe the motor strategies of typically developing infants. The AIMS is not intended to provide "cookbook" solutions for the treatment of infants with motor delays, but it permits therapists to identify the

missing components of a motor skill and develop appropriate intervention strategies.

Planning

At 4 months (corrected age), Amy was not able to maintain her head above 45 degrees in the prone position. From the description of the components of movement of this AIMS item *(Forearm Support 1)*, her therapist understood that to successfully accomplish this item Amy needed to bear weight on her upper chest, and her elbows had to be in line with her shoulders. Her therapist incorporated these positioning "cues" into her intervention suggestions.

EDUCATION (STUDENTS, PARENTS, AND CAREGIVERS)

The AIMS is used as an educational tool for physical and occupational therapy students who often have limited knowledge and experience with infant development. The AIMS item descriptors direct them to observe the components of motor skills that contribute to a specific motor milestone. Students learn to observe the underlying building blocks of each item, rather than taking a pass/fail approach to motor milestones. The observational approach of an AIMS assessment also encourages students to "learn from the infants," to appreciate the valuable information that may be gleaned from observing infants' spontaneous movements before extensive handling and examination of specific reflexes and muscle tone. Items describing the maturational sequence of motor milestones such as four-point kneeling, sitting, and creeping on hands and knees also provide students with ideas on how to encourage the maturation of these skills when working with infants with immature motor skills.

Parents and caregivers may also benefit from reviewing their infants' scoresheet with a therapist following an assessment. They easily see the skills that their infants currently have, the skills that will appear next, and how specific skills mature with development. Because the scoresheet has no age guidelines, the examiner is able to interpret and discuss an infant's scoring profile before discussing an infant's percentile rank.

Education

At each clinic visit Amy's therapist used the AIMS as a visual guide to discuss with Amy's parents the motor skills she had accomplished in prone, supine, sit, and stand and the skills that she would acquire next. The AIMS scoresheet represented a gross motor roadmap and helped them to understand the progression of gross motor milestones and what to do to encourage the progression of a motor milestone. For example, the first three stand items *(Supported Standing 1, Supported Standing 2, Supported Standing 3)* guided them to decrease their support of Amy's trunk in standing by moving their arms further down her trunk.

CONCLUSIONS

The use of the AIMS depends on the purpose of the assessment and the age and the motor abilities of the infant. While the AIMS has proven to be a strong discriminative index to identify an infant's present gross motor skills compared to a large normative sample, it should not be expected that an infant will retain the same percentile rank over serial assessments. The AIMS captures changes in an infant's abilities over time, but a statistical clinical minimally important difference has not been identified. The optimal circumstances to use the AIMS as a predictive index need further evaluation. The AIMS has been used successfully both for student education and enhancing parents' understanding of their infants' gross motor abilities.

REFERENCES

Albuquerque, P. L. De, Lemos, A., Guerra, M. Q. D. F., & Eickmann, S. H. (2015). Accuracy of the Alberta Infant Motor Scale (AIMS) to detect developmental delay of gross motor skills in preterm infants: A systematic review. *Developmental Neurorehabilitation, 18*(1), 15–21.

Aylward, G. P. (2009). Developmental screening and assessment: What are we thinking? *Journal of Developmental and Behavioral Pediatrics, 30*(2), 169–173.

Darrah, J., Piper, M. C., & Watt, M. J. (1998a). Assessment of gross motor skills of at-risk infants: Predictive validity of the Alberta Infant Motor Scale. *Developmental Medicine and Child Neurology, 40*, 485–491.

Darrah, J., Redfern, L., Maguire, T. O., Beaulne, A. P., & Watt, J. (1998b). Intra-individual stability of rate of gross motor development in full-term infants. *Early Human Development, 52*(2), 167–169.

Darrah, J., Senthilselvan, A., & Magill-Evans, J. (2009). Trajectories of serial motor scores of typically developing children: Implications for clinical decision making. *Infant Behavior and Development, 32*(1), 72–78.

Folio, M. R., & Fewell, R. R. (2000). *Peaboday developmental motor scales* (2nd ed.). Pro Ed.

Spittle, A. J., Doyle, L. W., & Boyd, R. N. (2008). A systematic review of the clinimetric properties of neuromotor assessments for preterm infants during the first year of life. *Developmental Medicine and Child Neurology, 50*(4), 254–266.

Spittle, A. J., Lee, K. J., Spencer-Smith, M., Lorefice, L. E., Anderson, P. J., & Doyle, L. W. (2015). Accuracy of two motor assessments during the first year of life in preterm infants for predicting motor outcome at preschool age. *PLoS ONE, 10*(5), 1–15.

10

Psychometric Properties of the AIMS

Thomas O. Maguire, PhD, Lynn Redfern, PhD

An important component of the development of any new instrument is the examination of its reliability and validity. Reliability can be defined as the consistency or reproducibility of scores obtained when the same group of individuals is assessed more than once with the same instrument. In the case of the Alberta Infant Motor Scale (AIMS), it was particularly important to document the reliability among different therapists when assessing the same infant and the reliability of scores obtained at two different points in time.

The validity of an instrument is the adequacy with which it measures the construct of interest. Although reliability is an essential aspect of validity, its presence is not sufficient evidence that the instrument covers the construct of interest—in this case, gross motor maturity. Assessment of validity should be thought of as a process whereby the instrument is subjected to investigations of its concurrent, structural, and discriminant characteristics. The concurrent validity of the AIMS was examined by comparing it to two widely used infant motor scales: the *motor scale* of the Bayley Scales of Infant Development (Bayley, 1969) and the *gross motor scale* of the Peabody Developmental Motor Scales (Folio & Fewell, 1983). Structural validity was examined through an analysis of the dimensionality and other scale properties of the AIMS and by documenting the ability of the instrument to discriminate between normal and abnormal development (the discriminant validity results are reported in Chapter 11).

SAMPLE AND DESIGN

The reliability and validity assessments were performed using data from 506 normal infants recruited through the Edmonton Board of Health baby clinics and meeting the following inclusion criteria:
- Gestational age of 38 to 42 weeks at the time of birth
- Birth weight of greater than 2500 g
- Uncomplicated delivery

- Deemed normal upon discharge from hospital
- No obvious abnormality at the time of assessment

The sample size was largely determined by the total number of items in the instrument, which is 58. A sample of approximately 500 infants was believed to be a reasonable compromise between a sufficient number of subjects to conduct a factor analysis and the costs of testing each infant.

The sample was age stratified, by month, through the first 18 months of life. The upper age limit of 18 months was chosen to be reasonably certain of capturing the age of independent walking in all normal infants. The instrument was constructed with the intent that it would be most sensitive around the middle of the first year of life, since that is generally considered to be the optimal time to identify infants who have a motor delay and to commence treatment programs for them. For this reason, slightly larger numbers of children were sampled in the age categories between 3 and 12 months than in the very young or older age categories.

Data were collected over a period of 15 months, beginning in December 1989 and ending in March 1991. Infants were assessed by one of six pediatric physical therapists who were experienced in infant motor assessment and trained in the administration of the AIMS.

The types of reliability and validity examined included interrater and test-retest reliability, concurrent validity with the Peabody and Bayley motor scales, and an extensive analysis of the scale properties of the new instrument. Thus the design required that some infants be tested by more than one rater and also tested on a second occasion. In addition, certain infants were simultaneously tested on the AIMS, the Peabody *motor scale*, and the Bayley *motor scale*. For the analysis of the instrument's scale properties, only one of these assessments was used, and in each case it was the initial AIMS assessment by the primary rater.

SCALE PROPERTIES OF THE AIMS

The scaling methods, which included tests of dimensionality and procedures for positioning items on the developmental continuum, were carried out with data from 479 infants who ranged in age from 0 to 15 months. Although the sample consisted of infants up to 18 months of age (n = 506), essentially all of the older infants had passed every item. As Wohlwill (1973) points out, "The scalability of any response matrix can be arbitrarily enhanced by ensuring a sufficiently large number of cases of subjects responding to or passing either all or none of the items, which necessarily constitute perfect scale patterns." He further indicates that this problem is most severe in the study of developmental sequences that concern only a limited portion of an age continuum. It was hoped that restricting the sample to only those infants expected to have some mixture of pass-fail scores would minimize this problem.

Tests of Dimensionality

Multidimensional scaling was the primary method for assessing the dimensionality of the data set. This was performed using a nonmetric procedure with ALSCAL (Young et al., 1978). The distance measure selected in the creation of the dissimilarities matrix for input into ALSCAL was the Euclidean distance for binary items. Goodness of fit indices were Kruskal stress value and the squared correlation between distances and dissimilarities. In accordance with Wohlwill's (1973) recommendation that dimensionality be tested both across and within age levels, multidimensional scaling was applied first to all data from infants 0 to 15 months of age and then to data from several individual age groups.

The multidimensional scaling results, using data from all 479 infants, indicated that a single dimension provides an excellent fit to these data, as evidenced by a stress value of 0.04 and RSQ of 0.995. To determine the nature of this dimension, the item scale values for the one-dimensional solution were examined in relation to the item order that was expected as a result of the content validation work and the feasibility study. With a few minor exceptions, the scale values for the one-dimensional solution were ordered in the manner expected. This suggests that the dimension is a developmental sequencing one and that the single construct underlying these data is gross motor maturity.

There was some concern that the one-dimensional model may have fit as well as it did because of the large variation in motor ability across the sample strata and the concomitant large variability across the item set in terms of the level of maturity required to perform the behaviors. Nunnally (1978) cautions that it is easy to fool oneself into believing that a unidimensional scale is present when one

takes a set of items widely dispersed in difficulty and administers them to a very diverse population. Also, Wohlwill (1973) emphasizes the importance of testing dimensionality both within and across age levels. For these reasons, the analyses were repeated using data within 3-month age groupings of infants.

The stress values for the one-dimensional solution ranged from 0.054 to 0.178, slightly higher than that obtained using all 479 infants. This finding probably reflects the fact that age (i.e., maturity) was the largest contributor to the variation among item scores. Grouping the data by age category removed much of the influence of age, with the result that the variance among items within age groups appears somewhat less systematic.

Still, for the majority of age groups, the stress values for the one-dimensional solution were very close to the two-dimensional stress values, which ranged from 0.003 to 0.106. Thus the conclusion that the scale is unidimensional was still deemed reasonable.

Dimensionality was also examined through nonlinear factor analysis, using the program NOHARM (Fraser & McDonald, 1988). The fit of a one-factor model was excellent, as determined by item loadings of 1 or near 1 on the single factor, very small unique variances, and a root mean square of residuals of 0.0174. Comparison with a two-factor nonlinear model was carried out by applying the Incremental Fit Index (De Champlain & Gessaroli, 1991). This involves comparing the residuals from the one-factor solution to the residuals from the two-factor solution. In this case, the fit index was zero, providing further strong evidence of unidimensionality.

Methods for Positioning Items

Nonmetric multidimensional scaling was the first model applied for the purposes of scaling the items, since it allowed the option of scaling on as many dimensions as were found to be necessary to adequately fit the data. The nonmetric approach had the advantage of producing scale values with interval level properties, while requiring only ordinal level assumptions about the relationships in the original data.

A second approach to item scaling was to examine item difficulty estimates derived according to various models. The method used first was a simple calculation of the proportion of infants passing each item, and this was obtained using the program LERTAP (Nelson, 1974). Next, a two-parameter item response model was applied to the data using the program LOGIST (Wingersky et al., 1982), and the item difficulty estimates were obtained.

Item difficulty estimates were then obtained from the NOHARM nonlinear factor analysis results. Further evidence as to the sequencing of items, as well as the actual distance between items on the age continuum, was gathered by examining the age at which 50% of infants passed each particular item. It was clear that the positioning of items was very similar, regardless of the scaling method used, and this provided convincing evidence of the validity of the item sequence.

Because the various models tested suggested almost identical item sequences, practical considerations such as ease of application and interpretability became the criteria for selecting a scaling model. By these criteria, multidimensional scaling seemed the most useful and thus was used to position the items on the final version of the AIMS.

SCORING SYSTEM

Following the determination of item sequence, the infants' test scores were derived according to two different scoring systems:

1. "Pass" scores were summed for each infant, giving a total number of items passed (range of 1–58).
2. Items were reordered, based on their multidimensional scale values, and a score was given to each infant corresponding to the position (1–58) of the highest item passed.

Each of these scoring systems had a certain appeal to the members of the research team. The "number of items passed" is the system used with most well-known motor scales and is very straightforward in its calculation. It also lends itself quite easily to the construction of norms tables, since typical total scores and ranges (or percentiles) can be reported for various age groups of infants. A total score or percentile rank is generally considered to be less problematic than certain other types of scores such as age equivalents, particularly when reporting an infant's performance to the parents.

The "highest item passed" system possesses the same advantages with regard to calculation, norming, and reporting. However, it has the added appeal of being a compensatory model for scoring, since it gives an infant credit for the level at which he or she is currently capable of performing, regardless of which behaviors were or were not performed previously. Thus the use of this system would avoid the situation of awarding "pass" scores for behaviors not actually observed but assumed to have been performed at an earlier time. It is also consistent with the opinion of many experts in infant motor assessment that it is the endpoint that is important in determining an infant's motor ability, rather than the means by which the infant arrived at that endpoint.

To evaluate the two scoring systems quantitatively, both types of scores were computed for all 506 infants. The correlation between the two scores was found to be 0.99, indicating a high degree of consistency across these two systems, when applied to data from normal infants. In addition, the infant's age had a strong relationship both with "number of items passed" (r – 0.95) and "highest item passed" (r = 0.94). These findings provided no real basis for choosing one scoring method over the other.

Through discussions within the research team, it was recognized that the consistency observed between the scoring methods might not hold when the instrument was applied to high-risk or abnormal infants. Specifically, it was felt that abnormal infants might pass certain items but be incapable of performing some earlier behaviors, particularly in a different postural position. This could give such an infant a higher score than was appropriate if scoring was based upon the highest item passed. For this reason, it was decided that the total number of items passed was a more reasonable scoring system to retain.

RELIABILITY

Overview

The reliability of the AIMS was examined in two ways. In the first, 253 infants were examined by two trained therapist assessors simultaneously. One of the assessors was designated as the "primary" assessor and was responsible for carrying out the actual assessment. The other assessor, the "observer" assessor, took a more passive role and observed the assessment as it proceeded, scoring the result independently of the first therapist. Comparison of the scores gives an indication of interassessor stability at one time. The second assessment occurred 3 to 7 days later, which was scheduled for each infant. In about one-third of the cases, this second assessment was done by a therapist who had not been involved either as primary assessor or observer with that infant. In about one-third of the cases, the primary assessor made the reassessment, and in the final third of the cases the observer assessor was used. Comparisons of the scores for the first analysis provide evidence about the joint effects of time and rater differences on the stability of ratings. The other two data sets give an indication of the effects of time on the stability of ratings. Because the infants' abilities change fairly rapidly, the influences of time are confounded with true growth or development. The time interval chosen was a compromise between making the time long enough so that the results of the first assessment would not influence the second to a great extent and the need to keep the interval short enough so that the infants' motor development had not changed substantially. In all, six assessors participated in the reliability study. Their involvement as primary, observer, and follow-up assessors was counterbalanced. However, to keep scheduling manageable, they were divided into two teams of three

TABLE 10.1 Reliability Plan

Time 1	Time 2	Type
Ab	C	3
Ab	A	1
Ac	B	3
Ac	C	2
Ba	C	3
Ba	A	2
Be	A	3
Be	B	1
Ca	B	3
Ca	C	1
Cb	A	3
Cb	B	2

A, B, C, Primary assessor; *a, b, c,* observer assessor; *type 1,*
primary rater over time; *type 2,* observer rater over time;
type 3, different rater—different time.

individuals. The assessment plan is shown in Table 10.1 for one of the teams. Approximately 40 infants did not return for the follow-up assessment.

The results were examined in several ways. Since the total score on the AIMS is used to estimate infant motor development, the main focus of the analyses was to provide estimates of reliability for total scores, both across and within age levels. Infants were selected for the reliability study to provide representation from birth to 17 months. For the purposes of these analyses, the age groups were clustered into four levels: birth through 3 months, 4 through 7 months, 8 through 11 months, and 12 months or older. There are two aspects to reliability that are important in the present context: First, the correlation between assessments

should be high; second, the difference between the means of the two sets of observations should be very small.

Interrater Reliabilities on One Occasion

The sample sizes, means, standard deviations, and correlations for total AIMS scores are shown in Table 10.2 for the total group and for each of the four age groups.

For the total score, the correlations between observers on a single occasion are very high, and the difference between the means of primary and observing assessors is very small. The standard error of measurement is about one item. In short, the instrument is very stable over raters at one time. Of course, the correlation for total scores is aided by the developmental trend that runs through the scale as shown in the various dimensional analyses. To see how stable the instrument is at various age levels, reliabilities and standard errors were calculated at each of the four levels. The lowest correlations occurred for the youngest and oldest children who are actually observed doing the fewest number of items. However, even here the reliabilities exceed 0.95. The reliabilities translate into standard errors of about 1 point for the youngest age group and for the infants in the 8- to 11-month-old group. The 4- to 7-month-old group has a standard error of about 1.4 items, and the oldest group has a standard error of 0.45. What all of this means in practical terms is that trained assessors can be used interchangeably to assess infants without increasing the error of measurement to an important extent.

Interrater Reliabilities Over Time

In Table 10.3, the reliabilities are shown for raters over time. For comparison purposes, the interassessor values for the total group are reproduced from Table 10.2. Type 1 reliabilities are based on the *primary* assessor being used on both occasions, type 2 reliabilities involve the *observing* assessor being used on both occasions, and type 3 reliabilities involve an assessor who had not previously seen the infant being used on the second occasion.

TABLE 10.2 Interrater Reliability Data for a Single Occasion

Sample	Primary Mean	Observer Mean	Primary SD	Observer SD	SE	Reliability	Sample Size
Total	34.73	34.66	18.65	18.63	1.01	0.9967	253
0–3 mo	10.12	9.93	4.26	4.07	0.86	0.9556	56
4–7 mo	26.57	26.65	8.05	8.00	1.38	0.9699	81
8–11 mo	48.56	48.37	8.26	8.32	1.11	0.9822	62
12 mo +	56.61	56.57	2.30	2.05	0.41	0.9588	54

TABLE 10.3   Interrater Reliability Data Across Occasions

Sample	First Mean	Second Mean	First SD	Second SD	SE	Reliability	Sample Size
One occasion	34.73	34.66	18.65	18.63	1.01	0.9967	253
Type 1	34.95	35.93	19.81	19.81	1.32	0.9556	56
Type 2	33.21	33.98	18.04	18.04	1.57	0.9925	56
Type 3	33.78	35.31	18.67	18.26	1.92	0.9891	98

For the three types of reliabilities calculated over time, the mean for the second occasion is about one item higher than the mean for the first occasion. Since the correlations are very high, it seems likely that the difference in means is largely due to real changes in infant performance. The differences between type 1 and type 2 reliability information are so small that for subsequent analyses no distinction was made between whether the rater at the first assessment was a primary or secondary assessor. The standard error of measurement that includes both occasion variation and between-rater variation is equivalent to about two items. Because it is larger than the values for types 1 and 2, it was decided to examine the effects of different raters over time for each of the age levels.

No distinction is made between primary and observer raters in Table 10.4, in which the results of the reliability analysis are presented for the effect of one rater on two occasions separated by up to 1 week. The results of the total sample are repeated to make comparisons easier.

The trend found in the total sample in which the second mean is about one item higher than the first mean continues with some variation at all age levels. This could be true growth coupled with the effect of the infant becoming more accustomed to the test setting on the second occasion. The reliabilities are all high except for the 25 infants in the oldest age group. Here, the infants are actually responding to relatively few items. For example, in the oldest age group the test is, in effect, a test of the standing items.

Consequently, the shortness of the instrument for the oldest group accounts for part of the relatively low reliability. The high means for the oldest infants arise from the scoring that assumes that the infant can perform (or could have performed) skills in the prone, supine, and sitting positions.

The results of the reliability study that confounds time with different assessors is shown in Table 10.5. Here the raters on each occasion are seeing the child for the first time.

Once again, the second observation results are generally higher than the first. The differences are slightly larger than those observed when the same rater was used over two times. At all ages, except the odd result at 4 to 7 months, the differences between raters over time were less than one item. The 2.7-item difference at 4 to 7 months does not yield to any simple explanation. The standard errors calculated in Table 10.5 are larger than those found in Table 10.4. These differences should be treated cautiously given the small sample sizes.

In interpreting scores at different age levels for a single administration of the AIMS, it might be useful to take the infant's observed score and add and subtract 1 standard error from it. This will produce an approximate 67% confidence band on the raw scores. Looking up the two ends of the confidence band on the table of percentiles provides an indication of how much the infant's score (expressed in percentile units) might be expected to vary from rater to rater. The results of using a confidence band may inject a healthy note of caution in the interpretation.

TABLE 10.4   Interrater Reliability Data Over Time (Same Assessor at Both Times)

Sample	First Mean	Second Mean	First SD	Second SD	SE	Reliability	Sample Size
Total	34.08	34.95	12.89	12.87	1.12	0.9925	112
0–3 mo	10.11	10.92	3.81	3.60	0.84	0.9485	26
4–7 mo	24.95	26.31	5.54	5.64	1.55	0.9230	36
8–11 mo	49.87	50.51	7.68	7.19	1.11	0.9775	25
12 mo +	56.36	56.84	1.43	1.36	0.53	0.8585	25

TABLE 10.5   Interrater Reliability Data Over Time (Different Assessor at Both Times)

Sample	First Mean	Second Mean	First SD	Second SD	SE	Reliability	Sample Size
Total	33.78	35.31	18.67	18.26	1.92	0.9891	98
0–3 mo	9.12	10.08	3.43	3.48	1.42	0.8245	24
4–7 mo	28	30.70	7.58	7.99	1.95	0.9267	30
8–11 mo	46.80	47.64	8.79	8.88	2.24	0.9352	25
12 mo +	56.36	56.89	1.79	2.18	0.74	0.8634	19

CONCURRENT VALIDITY

For the concurrent validity component, infants' total scores on the AIMS were correlated with the Peabody Developmental Motor Scale *gross motor* raw scores and with the *motor scale* of the Bayley Scales of Infant Development raw scores. These two scales were selected because they are the most widely used standardized infant motor scales. Although the limitations of these tools are widely recognized, it was seen as important to report how the new instrument compares with these established scales. Initially, it was anticipated that there would be a midrange correlation between the AIMS and each of these other scales. Very low correlations would be questionable because all three instruments are directed toward the general construct of emerging motor development. Similarly, very high correlations were not anticipated because the new instrument should provide more detailed information than either of the other two assessment scales.

One hundred and twenty infants were assessed by the same therapist on each of the three instruments. Only the 103 infants who were less than 13 months of age were included in the final analysis, since that is the typical age of independent walking, which represents the endpoint of the AIMS. Also, items beyond 13 months on the other two instruments capture behaviors not included within the AIMS, so validation against these more mature items was inappropriate.

Concurrent validity with the two established instruments was estimated with Pearson product-moment correlations, calculated first on all infants less than 13 months of age and then for three individual age groups. The correlations were as shown in Table 10.6.

Concurrent validity with both the *motor scale* of the Bayley Scales of Infant Development and the *gross motor scale* of the Peabody Developmental Motor Scales was also evaluated using 68 abnormal and at-risk infants. The sampling for this analysis is described in Chapter 11. The respective correlation coefficients are listed in Table 10.7.

TABLE 10.6   Concurrent Validity (Normal Infants)—Correlation Coefficients

0 to <13 months (n = 103):	
AIMS with Peabody	0.99
AIMS with Bayley	0.97
Peabody with Bayley	0.98
0 to <4 months (n = 23):	
AIMS with Peabody	0.90
AIMS with Bayley	0.84
Peabody with Bayley	0.93
4 to <8 months (n = 37):	
AIMS with Peabody	0.98
AIMS with Bayley	0.93
Peabody with Bayley	0.91
8 to <13 months (n = 43):	
AIMS with Peabody	0.94
AIMS with Bayley	0.85
Peabody with Bayley	0.92

TABLE 10.7   Concurrent Validity (Abnormal and At-risk Infants)—Correlation Coefficients

	Abnormal and At Risk (n = 68)	Abnormal (n = 20)	At Risk (n = 48)
Bayley	0.93	0.84	0.98
Peabody	0.95	0.87	0.98

The magnitude of these correlations, both for the total group and within each age group, and for the normal and abnormal infants, suggests very strong concurrent validity with the other two instruments. Given the evidence that all three instruments measure the same construct, one might question the need for a new instrument for assessing infant motor development. However, the ease of administration of the AIMS, along with the benefits of having a strictly observational assessment method, indicate that this instrument will meet a need not currently being met by existing instruments.

PREDICTIVE VALIDITY

Predictive validity of a screening instrument relates to its ability to correctly predict future performance of screened individuals on the outcome of interest. Future performance is measured by an accepted criterion or gold standard assessment.

Examination of predictive validity is approached through relating performance on the screening instrument to scores of the same subjects at the later assessment. In the case of the AIMS, the task was to see if it could accurately identify infants who at a later age will have a motor dysfunction.

The four indices to evaluate predictive validity are as follows:

1. Sensitivity—ability of the screening instrument to correctly identify true positives (e.g., infants who actually have motor dysfunction)
2. Specificity—ability of the screening instrument to correctly identify true negatives (e.g., infants who actually do not have motor dysfunction)
3. Positive predictive value (PPV)—probability that a given individual with a positive result on the screening test actually does have the condition (e.g., has motor dysfunction)
4. Negative predictive value (NPV)—probability that a given individual with a negative result on the screening test actually does not have the condition (e.g., does not have motor dysfunction)

The predictive validity examination of the AIMS (Darrah et al., 1998) was completed after publication of the first edition of *Motor Assessment of the Developing Infant*; a summary of their original work is provided here. Clinical challenges concerning prediction of infant motor performance are discussed in Chapter 9.

The purpose of the 1998 study was to identify cutoff scores on AIMS assessments of low birthweight infants (<1500 g; n = 164), at 4 and 8 months adjusted ages, that provided the best combination of predictive values for the infants' motor outcomes at 18 months adjusted age. A developmental pediatrician completed the outcome assessment, which included evaluation of posture, muscle tone, gross motor milestones, and reflexes. He classified each infant's outcome to one of three categories: Normal (N = 128), Suspicious (N = 14), or Abnormal (N = 22). Indices of predictive validity (sensitivity, specificity, negative and positive predictive values) of the AIMS were calculated using two different ways of categorizing the "suspicious" group of infants, grouping them with the normal infants in the first instance, and grouping them with the abnormal infants in the second. A "suspicious" category was necessary because at 18 months of age a final motor diagnosis of "normal" or "abnormal" is still challenging with some infants. To retain the effect of this "suspicious" group on predictive values, calculations were done two ways, placing infants in the "suspicious" group in the "normal" outcome category and then in the "abnormal" outcome category. Tables 10.8 and 10.9 summarize the predictive values by each of the two classification schemes.

As these findings demonstrate, the use of different possible cutoff points (AIMS percentile cutoffs) produced different effects on the sensitivity and specificity values. Higher percentile scores were associated with increased sensitivity and decreased specificity.

Darrah et al. (1998) discussed the challenges and implications inherent in balancing false-positive identification of normally developing infants as "abnormal," against false-negative identification of children with abnormal motor development as "normal." The authors concluded that the best compromise of sensitivity and specificity values was achieved using different AIMS percentile cutoffs at two ages: the 10th percentile at 4 months and the 5th percentile at 8 months.

CONCLUSIONS

The reliability and validity of the AIMS were examined following a thorough analysis of data collected on 506 Edmonton infants. It was concluded that the AIMS is a highly reliable instrument when used by different trained therapists and when applied to the same infants on two different occasions. In addition, there was compelling evidence that the instrument measures a single construct, gross motor maturity, and that its 58 items are appropriately sequenced along the developmental continuum. The high degree of congruence between AIMS scores and the Peabody and Bayley Infant Motor scores provided further evidence that the AIMS is a reliable and valid instrument for the measurement of infant motor development. In a later study (Darrah et al., 1998), the AIMS demonstrated good sensitivity and specificity in predicting motor performance of infants at 18 months of age.

TABLE 10.8 Predictive Validity Values for Abnormal vs Normal/Suspicious Category (N = 164)

	Cutoff (AIMS Centile)	Sens (%) (N = 22)	Spec (%) (N = 142)	+PV (%)	−PV (%)
4 Months					
	2nd	40.9	95.8	60.0	91.3
	5th	54.5	89.4	44.4	92.7
	10th	77.3	81.7	39.5	95.8
	16th	77.3	77.5	34.7	95.7
	25th	86.4	67.6	29.2	97.0
8 Months					
	2nd	72.7	94.4	66.7	95.7
	5th	86.4	93.0	65.5	97.8
	7th	90.9	91.5	62.5	98.5
	10th	90.9	85.9	50.0	98.4
	16th	95.5	82.4	45.7	99.2
	25th	100.0	63.4	29.7	100.0

Data from Darrah, J., Piper, M. C., & Watt, M. J. (1998). Assessment of gross motor skills of at-risk infants: Predictive validity of the Alberta Infant Motor Scale. *Developmental Medicine and Child Neurology, 40*(7), 485–491.

TABLE 10.9 Predictive Validity Values for Abnormal/Suspicious vs Normal Category (N = 164)

	Cutoff (AIMS Centile)	Sens (%) (N = 36)	Spec (%) (N = 128)	+PV (%)	−PV (%)
4 Months					
	2nd	30.6	96.9	73.3	83.2
	5th	41.7	90.6	55.6	84.7
	10th	58.3	82.8	48.8	87.6
	16th	58.3	78.1	42.9	87.0
	25th	72.2	69.5	40.0	89.9
8 Months					
	2nd	52.8	96.1	79.2	87.9
	5th	63.9	95.3	79.3	90.4
	7th	69.4	94.5	78.1	91.7
	10th	72.2	89.1	65.0	91.9
	16th	77.8	85.9	60.9	93.2
	25th	86.1	66.4	41.9	94.4

Data from Darrah, J., Piper, M. C., & Watt, M. J. (1998). Assessment of gross motor skills of at-risk infants: Predictive validity of the Alberta Infant Motor Scale. *Developmental Medicine and Child Neurology, 40*(7), 485–491.

REFERENCES

Bayley, N. (1969). *Bayley scales of infant development*. Institute of Human Development, University of California.

Darrah, J., Piper, M. C., & Watt, M. J. (1998). Assessment of gross motor skills of at-risk infants: Predictive validity of the Alberta Infant Motor Scale. *Developmental Medicine and Child Neurology, 40*(7), 485–491.

De Champlain, A. D., & Gessaroli, M. E. (1991). Assessing test dimensionality using an index based on nonlinear factor analysis. Paper presented at the American Educational Research Association Meeting, Chicago.

Folio, M. R., & Fewell, R. R. (1983). *Peabody developmental motor scales and activity cards: A manual*. DLM Teaching Resources.

Fraser, C., & McDonald, R. P. (1988). NOHARM: Least squares item factor analysis. *Multivariate Behavioral Research, 23*, 267–269.

Nelson, L. R. (1974). *Guide to LERTAP use and design computer program manual*. University of Otago, Education Department.

Nunnally, J. C. (1978). *Psychometric theory*. McGraw-Hill.

Wingersky, M. S., Barton, M. A., & Ford, F. M. (1982). *Logist user's guide*. Educational Testing Service.

Wohlwill, J. F. (1973). *The study of behavioral development*. Academic Press.

Young, F. W., Takane, Y., & Lewyckyj, Y. (1978). ALSCAL: A nonmetric multidimensional scaling program with several differences options. *Behavioral Research Methods Instrumentation, 10*, 451–453.

11

Norm Referencing of the Alberta Infant Motor Scale

Normative data provide details of the performance of the general population or specific populations so that an individual's performance may be compared with these norms (American Psychological Association, 1983). Because the Alberta Infant Motor Score (AIMS) was developed to identify those infants who exhibit delayed motor development, normative data are required to determine the individual infant's position with reference to a representative group of infants. Without additional interpretive data, a raw score on any test is meaningless. Norm-referenced test interpretation involves some method of assessing how an individual's raw test score compares with the scores of others in a similar group. In the case of the AIMS, an individual infant's test performance is interpreted by comparing it with the performance of a known group of age-matched Albertan infants. This known group is called the *normative sample*. The norms for the AIMS are recorded in a form of a table of equivalents between the *raw scores* (total AIMS score) and the *derived score* (percentile rank). The norms have been empirically established by determining how the infants in the normative sample scored on the AIMS. An infant's raw score is compared with the distribution of raw scores obtained by the normative sample to discover where the infant ranks in that distribution. The development of the AIMS normative data used to interpret an AIMS raw score and a subsequent reevaluation of these normative values are described in this chapter.

ORIGINAL NORMATIVE DATA

Normative Sample

A representative birth cohort of all infants born in the province of Alberta, Canada, between March 1990 and June 1992 constituted the original normative sample for the AIMS. The accessible population included *all*

infants—preterm, full term, and infants with congenital anomalies—who were born in Alberta between March 1990 and June 1992.

Alberta is a western province of Canada with a population of approximately 2.5 million people at the time of data collection. All health services in the province are provided through a government-financed national health insurance program. At the time of data collection community health services were delivered on a regional basis in 27 health units distributed geographically within the province.

To obtain a representative sample of all Albertan infants born over an 18-month period, a two-stage random sampling strategy was used with health units as the clusters. The final sample was to consist of 2400 infants stratified by age and sex. The average total number of births/year in Alberta at the time was approximately 42,445, distributed among the province's 27 health units as shown in Table 11.1. A map identifying the province's health units is seen in Fig. 11.1.

Edmonton and Calgary, as the two largest units, have about one-half of the province's births. Therefore one-half of the sample, or 1200 infants, was obtained through one randomly selected very large unit—Edmonton. The second 1200 infants were drawn from the remaining 25 health units using the following procedure: The health units were grouped into three levels—small, medium, and large—according to their number of births. The strata consisted of 9, 8, and 8 units, respectively. One-third of the health units were sampled from each stratum, and random samples of the sizes noted in Table 11.2 were drawn from each selected unit. The overall sampling fraction was 1/27, since the sampling time frame was 18 months.

Before sampling infants within units, the population of infants in each unit was stratified by sex and age. Equal numbers of male and female infants were included

TABLE 11.1   **Health Units—Total Births in 1989**

Health Unit (Unit No.)	Births
Edmonton (20)	10,502
Calgary (23)	12,107
East Central (9)	772
Athabasca (2)	672
Banff Park (27)	83
Barons-Eureka-Warner (3)	783
Big Country (5)	185
Chinook (17)	586
Lethbridge (24)	915
Drumheller (6)	528
West Central (8)	758
Foothills (10)	520
Fort-McMurray (16)	708
South Peace (22)	1,086
High Level–Fort Vermilion (1)	450
Jasper Park (25)	65
Leduc-Strathcona (19)	1,550
Southeastern Alberta (21)	1,191
Minburn-Vermilion (26)	376
Mount View (12)	1,066
North Eastern Alberta (7)	964
Peace River (4)	800
Red Deer Regional (18)	2,145
Stony Plain-Lac Ste. Anne (14)	1,131
Sturgeon (15)	1,523
Vegreville (13)	386
Wetoka (11)	593

within each age category so that separate norms could be developed for these two groups. The literature at the time documented small sex differences in early motor development, which justified the development of separate norms for boys and girls (Capute et al., 1985). The stratification by age for the total sample of infants is provided in Table 11.3. Because the largest number of items in the AIMS is contained within the 5- to 10-month age period, more infants of these ages were sampled than were infants of the younger or older ages. This procedure minimized the standard error

in the final normative tables for these very important age groups.

The total sample size of 2400 was chosen based on the distribution of age categories shown in Table 11.3. Our original intent was to report normative data for boys and girls separately, as well as to report norms for each age group. We believed that 75 to 100 infants in each of these sampling subgroups was the smallest acceptable number of infants upon which to report "representative" norms.

The Division of Vital Statistics, Department of Health, Province of Alberta provided a random sample of potential participants, according to the following criteria: (1) health unit, (2) sex, and (3) date of birth. Since all births in Alberta are registered with the Division of Vital Statistics within a few weeks of occurrence, this division had the most complete information available concerning the population of Alberta infants. It was standard practice in Alberta for the health units to be given immediate notification by the Division of Vital Statistics of the births occurring in their region.

Because Alberta's confidentiality guidelines precluded the release of infants' names to outside individuals, the lists of infants sampled within each health unit were forwarded from the Division of Vital Statistics to the appropriate health units. An initial telephone contact was made with the parents or guardians by health unit personnel. During this contact, the research was briefly described, and a verbal consent was sought to permit a member of the research team to make the contact. This second contact involved a more detailed explanation of the study, a request for written consent from the parent or guardian, and the scheduling of an appointment for the assessment. To offset those individuals who could not be reached or those individuals who would not consent to participate in the study, the Division of Vital Statistics randomly selected twice the number of infants required for each health unit. Despite this procedure, a final sample of 2202 infants, rather than the proposed 2400, participated in the norm-referencing study.

Each assessment was performed in the health unit by one of six physical therapists experienced in infant motor assessment and trained to an acceptable level of reliability (>.80) in the use of the AIMS.

Raw Scores and Derived Scores

Upon careful analyses of the normative data, no gender differences were documented in terms of performance on the AIMS. Table 11.4 presents a summary of the scores according to gender. Because of the lack of quantifiable gender differences, the scores for the entire sample were combined and analyzed according to age only.

The normative data collected on the total AIMS raw scores are presented in Appendix III. For each age month,

HEALTH UNITS OF ALBERTA

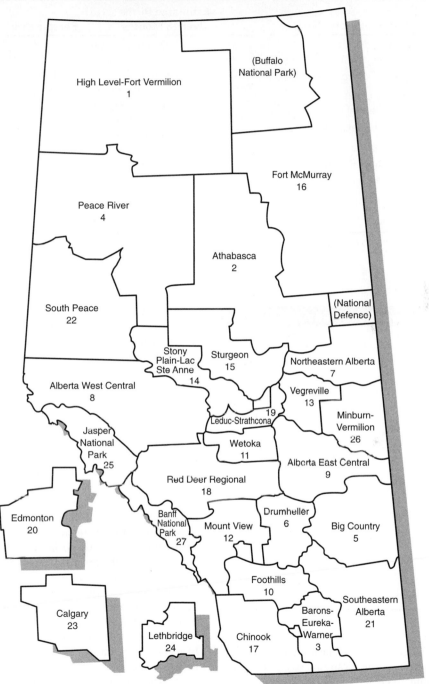

Fig. 11.1 Health units of Alberta, Canada.

TABLE 11.2 Sampling Design

	Unit Name (Unit No.)	Estimated Births Over 18 Months	Sample Size	Sampling Fraction
Small Units	Jasper Park (25)	97	10	$\frac{1}{3} \times \frac{1}{9}$
	Big Country (5)	278	31	
	High Level–Fort Vermilion (1)*	675	75	
Medium Units	Athabasca (2)	1008	112	$\frac{1}{3} \times \frac{1}{9}$
	West Central (8)	1125	125	
	Barons-Eureka-Warner (3)	1174	131	
Large Units	North Eastern (7)	1446	161	$\frac{1}{3} \times \frac{1}{9}$
	Southeastern (21)	1787	199	
	Red Deer Regional (18)	3217	356	
Very Large Units	Edmonton (20)	15,753	1200	$\frac{1}{2} \times \frac{1}{13}$
	TOTAL 10 Units		2400	

*This health unit was not able to participate in the project, and Minburn-Vermilion was randomly sampled from the group of small health units.

TABLE 11.3 Stratification by Age

Age of Infant	No. of Infants
1–2 mo	200
3–4 mo	200
5 mo	200
6 mo	200
7 mo	200
8 mo	200
9 mo	200
10 mo	200
11 mo	150
12 mo	150
13–14 mo	200
15–16 mo	150
17–18 mo	150

information is provided in terms of the numbers of infants sampled by sex, as well as the mean raw scores, standard deviations, and standard errors.

To ascertain more precisely the infant's exact position with reference to the normative sample, the total AIMS raw score (0–58) must be converted into some relative measure or derived score. These derived scores are designed to indicate an individual infant's relative standing in the normative sample and thus permit an evaluation of that infant's performance in reference to other age-matched infants.

Derived scores are based on a transformation of the raw score to some other unit of measurement that permits the comparison to the normative sample (Cermak, 1989). There are two ways that raw scores may be converted to derived scores: (1) developmental level attained or (2) relative position within a specified age group (Anastasi, 1988).

In age-equivalent norms, the infant's performance is compared with the performance of infants of many ages, and the resultant age-equivalent score gives an indication at what developmental or age level the infant is performing. For example, a 9-month-old infant who performs as well as the average 11-month-old infant could be described as having a motor performance age equivalence of 11 months.

In within-age group norms, the infant's performance is compared with the performance of the most nearly comparable group of infants in terms of age and then described in terms of the comparable group. For example, the performance of the same 9-month-old infant would be described in terms of other 9-month-old infants.

In the case of the AIMS, the derived scores are reported in terms of within-age group norms through the use of percentile ranks. A percentile rank indicates an individual infant's position relative to the age-matched normative sample. Percentile ranks are expressed in terms of the percentage of infants of a specified age in the normative sample whose scores fall below a given raw score. For example, if a total AIMS raw score of 15 corresponds to the 75th

TABLE 11.4 Comparison of Gender AIMS Scores by Age Group

Age Group (mo)	Gender	AIMS SCORE Mean	SD	t	p Value
0–<1	Boy	4.3	1.5	−0.78	0.44
	Girl	4.8	1.2		
1–<2	Boy	7.1	1.9	−0.70	0.49
	Girl	7.5	2		
2–<3	Boy	9.9	2.5	0.32	0.75
	Girl	9.7	2.4		
3–<4	Boy	12.4	2.9	−0.45	0.66
	Girl	12.8	3.7		
4–<5	Boy	18	4.2	0.40	0.69
	Girl	17.7	4.1		
5–<6	Boy	23.1	4.6	−0.28	0.78
	Girl	23.3	4.9		
6–<7	Boy	28.5	5.4	0.49	0.63
	Girl	28.1	5.7		
7–<8	Boy	32.6	6.9	0.66	0.51
	Girl	31.9	6.8		
8–<9	Boy	39.2	8.6	−0.96	0.34
	Girl	40.3	8.8		
9–<10	Boy	46.4	6.8	1.75	0.08
	Girl	44.5	8.1		
10–<11	Boy	49.1	6.1	−0.44	0.66
	Girl	49.5	5.7		
11–<12	Boy	51.5	6.4	0.46	0.64
	Girl	51	7.8		
12–<13	Boy	54.3	4.4	−0.63	0.53
	Girl	54.8	4.6		
13–<14	Boy	55.6	4.6	−0.02	0.98
	Girl	55.6	5.5		
14–<15	Boy	57.3	1.3	1.68	0.10
	Girl	56.4	2.6		
15–<16	Boy	57.7	0.6	−1.97	0.06
	Girl	57.9	0.2		
16–<17	Boy	57.8	0.6	−0.37	0.71
	Girl	57.8	0.4		
17–<18	Boy	57.9	0.3	0.81	0.42
	Girl	57.8	0.4		
18–<19	Boy	57.6	0.5	−0.72	0.48
	Girl	57.8	0.8		

percentile for 3-month-old infants, it means that 75% of 3-month-old infants had raw scores of 15 or less. Similarly, a 3-month-old infant with a score of 15 scored as well as or better than 75% of the 3-month-old infants in the normative sample. With percentiles, the lower the percentile, the less mature the infant's motor development.

The percentile ranks for the total AIMS scores according to age are presented in Appendix II and Appendix IV. Appendix II presents the appropriate percentile ranks associated with every possible total AIMS score by age groupings. These percentile ranks have been determined by calculating the appropriate z-scores (based on the means and standard deviations for the respective age groupings) for each total score. For example, a 6.5-month-old infant who obtains a total AIMS score of 27 is at the 40th percentile for age. Because the percentile ranks listed in Appendix II have been averaged over the entire age month, it is important to recognize that the listed percentiles are less accurate for infants whose age at the time of testing falls at either end of the age month, such as an infant who is 6 months and 2 days or an infant who is 6 months and 28 days old.

Appendix IV provides the total AIMS scores according to age associated with six percentile rankings—that is, the 5th, 10th, 25th, 50th, 75th, and 90th percentiles for each age group of infants. This appendix essentially replicates the developmental graph found in Appendix I that visually depicts the six percentile rankings in graph form. A child's individual total AIMS score may be placed on the developmental graph according to age. The total AIMS score also may be placed between the appropriate percentile rankings as listed in Appendix IV to provide the examiner with an estimate of the percentile ranking of the infant. For example, an infant who is between 4 and 5 months of age and obtains a score of 19 is performing between the 50th and 75th percentiles for age.

Application of Normative Data—Case Validation Study

The normative data generated for the AIMS were applied in a case validation study. The basic assumption was made, using the means and standard deviations of the total AIMS scores obtained for each age group, that infants who obtained scores that fell between −1 SD and −2 SD from the mean for a specific age group exhibited "suspicious" motor performance. Similarly, infants who obtained scores that fell below −2 SD from the mean exhibited "abnormal" motor performance (Fig. 11.2).

Although the use of −1 SD and −2 SD as cutoff points to classify infants as suspicious and abnormal is accepted practice with developmental scales, this statistical approach to abnormality, using the properties of normal distribution, may be inappropriate for classifying infants' motor abilities. Motor skills are not categorically abnormal or normal; rather a continuum of severity exists. Predictive abilities might be improved by evaluating a range of cutoff points on a test and choosing the score with the most acceptable combination of sensitivity, specificity, and negative and positive predictive values as the positivity criterion. The age of the infant, the degree of abnormality to be detected, and the consequences of both false-positive and false-negative results should all be considered when assigning cutoff scores. A predictive validity study conducted after publication of this book evaluated a range of cutoff scores for the AIMS (Darrah et al., 1998). It is summarized in Chapter 10. In the case validation study, two groups of infants were assessed using the AIMS: 18 infants with a definitive diagnosis of

Classification Criteria

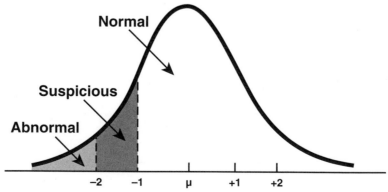

Fig. 11.2 Use of normative data obtained from the AIMS in a case validation study.

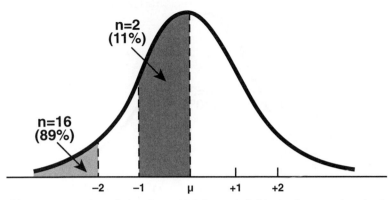

Case Validation – Abnormal Babies
(n = 18)

n=2
(11%)

n=16
(89%)

−2   −1   μ   +1   +2

Fig. 11.3 Graphic representation of data from 18 infants definitively diagnosed as having abnormal motor development.

abnormal motor development and 44 infants who were at risk for motor disorders because of either a gestational age of less than 32 weeks or term asphyxia. Therapists who performed the assessments were unaware of the infants' developmental status and birth history. The results of these assessments were compared with the normative data.

Of the 18 diagnosed abnormal infants, 16 (89%) were considered "abnormal" on the basis of their AIMS scores—that is, they received scores lower than 2 SD below the mean for their respective ages. Two infants obtained "normal" scores. The diagnoses of the two abnormal infants who were deemed to be developing normally on the AIMS were Erb palsy and lipomatous meningomyelocele (Fig. 11.3).

Of the 44 at-risk infants, 10 (23%) were considered to be "suspicious" (between 1 SD and 2 SD below the mean) and 3 (7%) were considered to be "abnormal" (>2 SD below the mean) (Fig. 11.4). Although the final diagnoses of the at-risk infants were not known, the findings agreed with the majority of studies at the time that suggested that approximately 25% to 30% of at-risk infants exhibited some form of neuromotor disturbance early in life (Coolman et al., 1985; Piper et al., 1988). The findings of this case validation suggested that the AIMS is able to accurately discriminate, at the time of testing, those children with abnormal motor development from those who exhibit normal motor development. In addition, the AIMS is able to categorize at-risk infants in the first 18 months of life into three categories: those infants who at the time of testing are exhibiting suspicious patterns of motor development from those who have abnormal or normal patterns of movement. However, −1 SD and −2 SD are not recommended as cutoffs on the

AIMS to predict the future gross motor outcome of individual infants since these cutoffs may result in a high false-positive rate of identification.

REEVALUATION OF THE NORMATIVE DATA

A reevaluation of the normative data was undertaken for three reasons: (1) concern that some prone items may occur later than the ages represented in the original norms because of the increased practice of placing an infant in the supine sleep position recommended in Back to Sleep campaigns (Kattwinkel et al., 1992), (2) the normative data did not represent the increased ethnic diversity in the Canadian population, and (3) the concern that the AIMS norms were not applicable to other countries (Fleuren et al., 2007). The methods and results are summarized here; further information is available in the original publication (Darrah et al., 2014).

A cross-sectional cohort study design was used for the reevaluation project. In the original normative study, the 58 AIMS items were placed in one of three age groups representing their ages of emergence: 22 weeks or less (19 items), 23 to 36 weeks (19 items), and 37 weeks and older (20 items). For the reevaluation study, a sample of 450 infants (150 in each age category) would produce a standard error equal to the largest standard error in the original AIMS normative data. An additional 75 infants were included in each age category in the recruitment strategy to ensure that the sample captured the variability of the appearance of infant motor skills and the ethnic diversity of the Canadian population. Assuming a 25% attrition rate, the recruitment target was 845 infants. This target was

Case Validation – At-risk Babies
(n = 44)

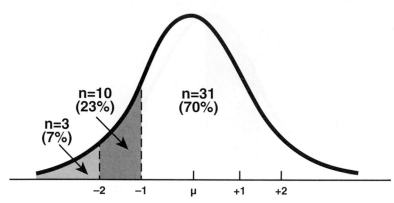

Fig. 11.4 Graphic representation of data from 44 infants at risk for motor disorders.

achieved; 868 infants were recruited and 650 infants (338 males, 312 females) completed an assessment.

Families were recruited when their infants were born in hospitals in six Canadian cities. Each infant was randomly assigned an assessment age in one of the three age categories. All infants had one assessment at their assigned age between 2 weeks and 18 months (adjusted age for preterm infants). Two pediatric therapists in each of the six cities attended an initial 1-day training session to do AIMS assessments. During the study they also participated in three teleconferences to discuss assessment procedures as they assessed older infants. To ensure interrater reliability, the assessors achieved an 80% item agreement with the trainer in the scoring of video-recorded AIMS assessments on three different occasions. The two trainers evaluated assessment standardization by doing site visits to observe each therapist completing an assessment with an infant. To standardize scoring, each therapist scored the individual items, and two project coordinators calculated the infants' total score and percentile rank using the normative graph (see Appendix I).

The original and the contemporary data were compared by using a logistic regression method to compare the ages when 50% of the infants in each data set achieved each item on the AIMS (item location). This analytic strategy allowed comparison of the two data sets without recruiting a new sample as large as the original normative sample. This strategy may be replicated by other researchers interested in comparing the scores of their infant populations to the AIMS norms.

Forty-three items were used in the final analyses. Comparison of the data sets revealed that most of the items differed by 2 weeks or less at the age when 50% of the

infants passed an item. The average age difference between item locations was less than 0.7 week (Table 11.5).

The normative age values from the original data set, when converted to the contemporary scale, differed by less than 1 week. Since the percentile graph values are presented in 1-week age intervals, the results of the re-norming study suggest that the percentile rank of individual infants would remain essentially the same using the analyses from the contemporary data and that the original normative data are still appropriate. A full description of the re-norming analysis approach is available in the supporting information provided with the original publication (Darrah et al., 2014).

CONCLUSION

The AIMS is a norm-referenced test based on age- and sex-stratified normative data collected on a representative sample of 2202 infants. A reevaluation of the normative data confirmed that the original normative information remains appropriate to interpret an AIMS raw score. The results of a predictive validity study suggested that cutoff scores of the 10th percentile at 4 months of age and the 5th percentile at 8 months of age resulted in the best combination of sensitivity and specificity values (Darrah et al., 1998). If other cutoff points are considered in clinical practice, it is important to evaluate their predictive values.

Parents may need guidance from the examiner to interpret an AIMS percentile score. They often assume that percentile ranks represent the percentage of correct AIMS items passed for their infant's age, and they are disappointed and often concerned if their infant scores are below the 50th percentile because they view it as "below average."

TABLE 11.5   Agreement Between Item Locations for 43 Items Used in Conversion Equation

Difference in Location	Number of Items	Item Location Is Earlier in Original Data	Item Location Is Earlier in Contemporary Data
<1 week	21	15	6
1–2 weeks	11	8	3
2–3 weeks	9	8	1
3–4 weeks	1	0	1
4–5 weeks	1	1	0
Total	**43**	**32**	**11**

Darrah, J., Bartlett, D., Maguire, T., Avison, W., & Lacaze-Masmonteil, T. (2014). Have infant gross motor abilities changed in 20 years? A re-evaluation of the Alberta Infant Motor Scale normative values. *Developmental Medicine and Child Neurology, 56*(9), 877–881.

They need to be reassured that 50% of the infants in the normative sample in the same age category as their infant received scores lower than their infant, and that the majority of these infants had typical gross motor abilities. Interpretation of a percentile rank score is often not intuitive. An infant's AIMS percentile rank should not be used in isolation to make clinical decisions regarding follow-up or intervention. Rather it should be used in conjunction with other sources of information such as the infant's medical history, other medical testing, and parents' concerns.

REFERENCES

American Psychological Association. (1983). *Standards for educational and psychological tests.* American Psychological Association.

Anastasi, A. (1988). *Psychological testing* (6th ed.). Macmillan.

Capute, A. J., Shapiro, B. K., Palmer, F. B., Ross, A., & Wachtel, R. C. (1985) Normal gross motor development: The influences of race, sex and socio-economic status. *Developmental Medicine & Child Neurology, 27,* 635–643.

Cermak, S. (1989). Norms and scores. In L. J. Miller (Ed.), *Developing norm-referenced standardized tests* (pp. 91–123). Haworth Press.

Coolman, R. B., Bennett, R. C., Sells, C. J., Swanson, M., Andrews, M., & Robinson, N. (1985). Neuromotor development of graduates of the neonatal intensive care unit: Patterns encountered in the first two years of life. *Journal of Developmental and Behavioral Pediatrics, 6,* 327–333.

Darrah, J., Bartlett, D., Maguire, T., Avison, W., & Lacaze-Masmonteil, T. (2014). Have infant gross motor abilities changed in 20 years? A re-evaluation of the Alberta Infant Motor Scale normative values. *Developmental Medicine and Child Neurology, 56*(9), 877–881.

Darrah, J., Piper, M. C., & Watt, M. J. (1998). Assessment of gross motor skills of at-risk infants: Predictive validity of the Alberta Infant Motor Scale. *Developmental Medicine and Child Neurology, 40*(7), 485–491.

Fleuren, K. M. W., Smit, L. S., Stijnen, T., & Hartman, A. (2007). New reference values for the Alberta Infant Motor Scale need to be established. *Acta Paediatrics, 96*(3), 424–427.

Kattwinkel, J., Brooks, J., & Myerberg, D. (1992). Positioning and SIDS. *Pediatrics, 89*(6), 1120–1126.

Piper, M. C., Mazer, B., Silver, K. M., & Ramsay, M. (1988). Resolution of neurological symptoms in high-risk infants during the first two years of life. *Developmental Medicine & Child Neurology, 30,* 26–35.

Percentile Ranks—AIMS Scores

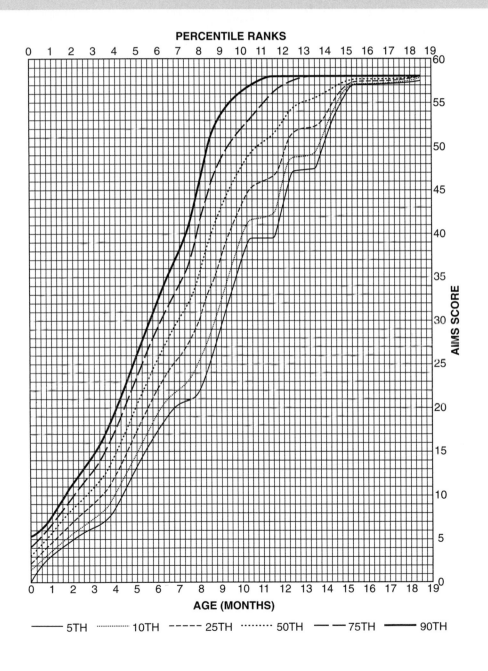

Percentile Ranks by Age Grouping

Percentile Ranks by Age Grouping

Raw Score	≥0	1	2	3	4	5	6	7	8	9	10	11	12	13	14
													Age in Months (mid-month)		
1	1														
2	3														
3	14	1													
4	36	4	1												
5	64	12	2	1											
6	86	25	6	2											
7	97	43	12	5											
8	99	63	23	8	1										
9		80	37	14	2										
10		91	53	22	3										
11		97	69	31	5										
12		99	82	43	8	1									
13			91	55	12	2									
14			96	67	17	3									
15			98	77	24	4									
16			99	85	32	6	1								
17				91	41	10	2	1							
18				95	51	14	3	2							
19				97	60	19	5	3							
20				99	69	25	7	4	1						
21					77	32	9	5	2						
22					84	40	13	7	2						
23					89	48	17	9	3						
24					93	57	22	11	4						
25					96	65	27	15	5						
26					97	72	34	18	6						
27					99	79	41	22	7						
28						84	48	27	9						
29						89	55	32	11	1					
30						92	62	37	13	2					
31						95	69	43	16	3					
32						97	75	40	19	4					
33						98	81	54	22	5					
34						99	85	60	26	6					
35							80	66	29	8	1	1			
36							92	71	33	10	1	2			
37							94	76	38	13	2	2			
38							96	80	42	16	3	3			
39							97	84	46	19	4	4			
40							98	89	51	23	6	6			
41							99	90	56	27	8	8			
42								92	60	32	11	10			
43								94	64	37	14	12			
44								96	69	42	18	15	1	1	
45								97	73	47	23	19	2	2	
46								98	76	52	29	23	3	3	
47								98	80	58	35	27	5	4	
48								99	83	63	41	32	7	6	
49									86	68	48	38	11	9	
50									88	73	54	43	15	13	
51									90	77	61	48	21	18	
52									92	81	67	54	28	24	1
53									94	84	73	60	36	30	2
54									95	87	79	65	45	37	7
55									96	90	83	70	54	45	17
56									97	92	87	75	62	53	32
57									98	94	90	79	70	61	52
58									>98	>95	>93	>83	>77	>68	>71

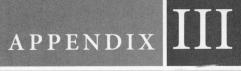

Normative Data

Normative Data

Age (mo)	Male	Female	Total	Mean	SD	SE
0–<1	13	9	22	4.5	1.37	0.19
1–<2	27	29	56	7.3	1.96	0.27
2–<3	60	58	118	9.8	2.42	0.34
3–<4	45	45	90	12.6	3.29	0.46
4–<5	69	53	122	17.9	4.15	0.58
5–<6	80	109	189	23.2	4.75	0.67
6–<7	119	106	225	28.3	5.50	0.77
7–<8	120	102	222	32.3	6.85	0.96
8–<9	109	111	220	39.8	8.69	1.22
9–<10	105	84	189	45.5	7.47	1.05
10–<11	81	74	155	49.3	5.92	0.83
11–<12	77	78	155	51.3	7.11	1
12–<13	53	71	124	54.6	4.52	0.63
13–<14	47	39	86	55.6	5.01	0.7
14–<15	36	25	01	56.9	1.97	0.28
15–<16	10	21	40	57.8	0.45	0.06
16–<17	28	21	49	57.8	0.55	0.08
17–<18	28	21	49	57.9	0.35	0.05
18–<19	14	16	30	57.7	0.64	0.09

Percentile Ranks

Percentile Ranks

Age (mo)	5th	10th	25th	50th	75th	90th
0–<1	2.2	2.7	3.6	4.5	5.4	6.3
1–<2	4.1	4.8	6	7.3	8.6	9.8
2–<3	5.8	6.7	8.2	9.8	11.4	12.9
3–<4	7.2	8.4	10.4	12.6	14.8	16.8
4–<5	11.1	12.6	15.1	17.9	20.7	23.2
5–<6	15.4	17.1	20	23.2	26.4	29.3
6–<7	19.3	21.2	24.6	28.3	32	35.4
7–<8	21	23.5	27.7	32.3	36.9	41.1
8–<9	25.5	28.7	33.9	39.8	45.7	50.9
9–<10	33.2	35.9	40.5	45.5	50.5	55.1
10–<11	39.6	41.7	45.3	49.3	53.3	56.9
11–<12	39.6	42.2	46.5	51.3	56.1	58
12–<13	47.2	48.8	51.6	54.6	57.6	58
13–<14	47.4	49.2	52.2	55.6	58	58
14–<15	53.7	54.4	55.6	56.9	58	58
15–<16	57.1	57.2	57.5	57.8	58	58
16–<17	56.9	57.1	57.4	57.8	58	58
17–<18	57.3	57.5	57.7	57.9	58	58
18–<19	56.6	56.9	57.3	57.7	58	58

INDEX

Note: Page numbers in *italics* indicate figures; those followed by t indicate tables.